D1483131

B**A**D BLOOD

THE TRAGEDY OF THE CANADIAN
TAINTED BLOOD SCANDAL

173102107

Vic Parsons

WITHDRAWN

...ITY OF
...A COLLEGE
...SOURCE CENTRE
KING CAMPUS

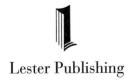

Lester Publishing

To David, and to all the others affected by this tragedy, this book is dedicated.

Copyright © 1995 by Vic Parsons

All rights reserved. No part of this work covered by the copyrights hereon may be reproduced or used in any form or by any means — graphic, electronic or mechanical, including photocopying, recording, taping or information storage and retrieval systems — without the prior written permission of the publisher or, in the case of photocopying or other reprographic copying, a licence from the Canadian Copyright Licensing Agency. Lester Publishing Limited acknowledges the financial assistance of the Canada Council, the Ontario Arts Council, and the Ontario Publishing Centre.

CANADIAN CATALOGUING IN PUBLICATION DATA

Parsons, Vic, 1942-
  Bad blood : the tragedy of the Canadian tainted blood scandal

ISBN 1-895555-51-5

1. Blood banks — Canada — Quality control.
I. Title.

RM171.P37   1995   362.1'784'0971   C95-930153-4

Lester Publishing Limited
56 The Esplanade
Toronto, Ontario
Canada M5E 1A7

Printed and bound in Canada

95 96 97 98   5 4 3 2 1

CONTENTS

Blood Products from Donor to Recipient

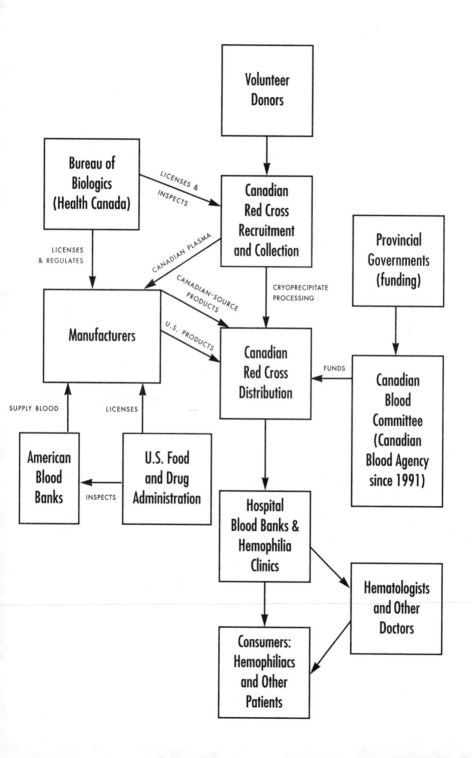

THE MAIN PLAYERS

The **Canadian Red Cross Society** was asked by the federal government in 1941 to set up a civilian blood service. It recruits donors, collects blood at collection centres and mobile clinics, sends plasma to manufacturers for fractionation, and distributes the products. The Red Cross also processes a clotting factor known as cryoprecipitate from fresh-frozen plasma.

The **Bureau of Biologics** is a division of the federal Health Protection Branch that regulates biological drugs, including blood and blood products, vaccines, and other drugs made from animal or human sources. It inspects and licenses Red Cross centres and conducts on-site checks of manufacturers. In its own words, the Bureau's responsibility is to "ensure safe and efficacious biological drugs are available to the Canadian public, which is accomplished through evaluation, licensing, inspection, and lot-by-lot approvals."

The **Canadian Blood Committee** (CBC) was set up in 1981 and included representatives of the federal government and each of the provinces. Its role was to fund the blood products obtained and distributed by the Red Cross. It had an advisory sub-committee which provided a forum for discussion of the blood crisis in the late 1980s.

The committee was replaced in April 1991 by the **Canadian Blood Agency** (CBA), an incorporated non-profit organization of the provinces and territories (it excludes the federal government). The Agency has a mandate to "direct the Canadian blood system."

The manufacturers, or "fractionators," are private companies that produce and sell an assortment of blood derivatives.

The only significant Canadian manufacturer was **Connaught Laboratories**, which stopped making Factor VIII concentrates in the late 1980s after severe production problems that forced larger-than-expected imports of American-made products.

The most important U.S. supplier is **Cutter Laboratories**, sometimes referred to as **Miles-Cutter**, which for several years has fractionated Canadian-source plasma. Others are U.S. firms **Armour, Baxter** (which has **Hyland** and **Travenol** divisions), **Alpha Therapeutics**, and Austria-based **Immuno**.

The **Canadian Hemophilia Society** (CHS) is the national volunteer organization representing an estimated 2,500 Canadian hemophiliacs. It has also taken on some responsibilities for persons infected with HIV through blood transfusions, although there is also an HIV-Tranfused (HIV-T) group that has split from the Society. Each province has a chapter of the CHS—for example, **Hemophilia Ontario.**

The **Medical and Scientific Advisory Committee** (MSAC) is a group of professionals, mostly hematologists or other physicians, who have provided counsel to the volunteer society. Many representatives in the MSAC are also associated with the Red Cross.

Some hospitals in major cities have comprehensive hemophilia clinics, where patients can go for regular monitoring, treatment, information, and advice. A complete clinic may provide medical, dental, physiotherapy, counselling, and, today, specific care for people with AIDS.

Hemophiliacs usually pick up their clotting factors from hospital blood banks.

Other groups and organizations play lesser roles in the story of tainted blood in Canada, but these are the principal actors.

ACKNOWLEDGEMENTS

Early in 1994, a woman I will call Sarah died. I can't say I really knew Sarah. But hearing of her death left me with a profound impression of how many people have touched the creation of this book.

In September 1992, Sarah appeared on a panel with my wife, Lorraine, and me at a Canadian Hemophilia Society retreat at Orillia, Ontario. Sarah, who sat beside me on the panel, had become HIV-positive through a blood transfusion. She spoke first, telling her story to the audience quietly, with dignity, inevitably with great feeling. I felt like reaching out and touching her as a sign of solidarity, but I held back.

When it was our turn, and I had to speak, the emotion welled up and I was struggling. I felt Lorraine's hand on my neck, but then there was another hand, Sarah's, on my elbow, both giving the support I needed to carry through. As we pull ourselves through this catastrophe, we need the comfort of those around us — be they relatives, friends, or strangers.

I've been given much active support while I was working on the book and always, when things got tough, there was the inspiration derived from the courage of others. I am in awe of some of those often unsung heroes. I think particularly of John Meyers, who came to

Ottawa from southwestern Ontario in 1993 to demonstrate for the new blood products he would never benefit from. John had no immune system left, but he took on the extra stress of appearing before the Canadian Blood Agency. John died within weeks, leaving a legacy — those products are now standard treatment in Canada.

There have been so many others besides John and Sarah — friends, relatives, workmates, and activists — that I couldn't possibly thank them all by name. These are people who offered suggestions and ideas, forced me to think of the work in progress, and provided information, much of it personal.

No one can undertake a book on this subject without relying heavily on the impressive archival work put together for the Canadian Hemophilia Society's compensation battle in the 1980s by Bob Gibson, Stephen Christmas — both of whom have died in this tragedy — and others. I'd like particularly to thank the staff and executive of Hemophilia Ontario; Santo Caira, formerly of the Toronto-Central Ontario Hemophilia Society; Bob O'Neill of St. Paul's Hospital in Vancouver; the CHS's David Page, Lindee David, Bob Pedersen, and Elaine Woloschuk; the family of Eva Blaikie; Jerry Freise; and many others who contributed. Thanks are due to my agent, Larry Hoffman, who believed in the book; Malcolm Lester, who saw the significance of the story; and my editor, Meg Taylor, and the proofreader, Alison Reid, who beat it into shape.

Then there's my daughter Jill, wise beyond her years, who represents the future of health consumer groups like the Canadian Hemophilia Society. At age fifteen, she bravely argued for new blood products before an imposing group of senior provincial bureaucrats, and prevailed.

I must give credit to David, of whom I am most proud, a son who has never been afraid to live life to the fullest, and who has had a deep effect on everyone who has crossed his path.

Most of all, I want to thank Lorraine, who really gave birth to this book, urging me on when I became discouraged, and compelling me to face the reality of our lives.

INTRODUCTION

Blood evokes images of life, kinship, courage, guilt, anger, and death. It is thought to resemble the primordial soup from which life emerged on earth. A salty, protein- and mineral-rich medium, blood teems with living cells — cellular matter originating from the organism itself — side by side with hostile aliens that could threaten the host's existence. Blood cleanses the body of unwanted corruption, carries oxygen to the brain and nourishment to the cells, and fights off intruders. It flows within all higher animals like a vestige of our brine-soaked creation.

The human body contains about 5.5 litres of blood. About half the volume of blood is plasma, a fluid that includes a wide variety of proteins, and most of the balance is blood cells — white cells, red cells, and platelets. Sodium, potassium, calcium, magnesium, chlorides, and bicarbonate are among the ions present. Sugars, amino and fatty acids, hormones, carbon dioxide, oxygen, and nitrogen-bearing wastes complete the makeup of this internal sea.

Our modern word is virtually unchanged from the word "blod," used a thousand years ago in Old English. Some believe the root is connected to the word "bloom," meaning brightness of colour. When someone is quick to anger, we call them hot-blooded. The indignant person may growl that an injustice makes the blood boil. Calculating villains commit crimes in cold blood. Bloodhounds are used to track down fugitives, supposedly following the scent of their blood. A bloodless wretch lacks spirit. The word "leech" comes from the old Anglo-Saxon word for physician — someone who bled the patient to suck toxins from the body.

All over the world, blood is associated with the life force. The Koran invokes "the name of your Lord who created — created man from clots of blood." The *Huai-nan Tzu*, an early Chinese Taoist text, tells us: "The blood and vital breath are the flowerings of mankind." D. H. Lawrence says: "That I am part of the earth my feet know perfectly, and my blood is part of the sea." "Blood's a rover," wrote A. E. Housman.

There is kinship and unity in blood. We speak of royal blood, blue bloods, pure blood, blood relatives, and blood lines. Blood is thicker than water, the English proverb goes. Shakespeare's Henry V, on the field of battle, vowed that those who shed their blood with him would forever be his brothers. St. Paul wrote that Christ "hath made of one blood all nations."

The spilling of blood is a heinous crime that demands justice. "The voice of thy brother's blood crieth unto me from the ground," the Book of Genesis rumbles. "Oh God! that bread should be so dear, And flesh and blood so cheap!" wails Thomas Hood. Blood money is paid the next of kin as appeasement during blood feuds.

And Bad Blood means that something has gone terribly wrong in a relationship.

In the fall of 1993, a group of ten people were spread out over the living-room floor of my Ottawa home, engrossed in the work of hand-sewing the names of eight dead men on a memorial quilt. The names and faces of most of the deceased were familiar to me, and though none were close friends, I still recall them — Michel, Frank, Eric, Brian, Denis, John, Marc, and David. Unfortunately, someone said, the quilt — which included a little reminder of each — would continue to grow. It was a cruel reality.

All of these men and at least a thousand other Canadians—perhaps many more—were infected in the early to mid-1980s with the human immunodeficiency virus (HIV) through the blood supply. The tragic irony of this infection was that the blood transfused into the veins of those unfortunate patients was intended to give life. Instead, it has brought premature death to hundreds of Canadians. Hundreds more must come to grips with the likelihood of an early demise, all the while trying to retain some sense of dignity in the tragedy.

Canadian hemophiliacs and their families were the first and hardest hit by the tainted blood. Sometimes described as the "miner's canaries," an early-warning line for the blood system, nearly half of the country's hemophiliacs were infected with the virus that ultimately causes AIDS. Some unwittingly infected their spouses, and in a few cases, babies in the womb.

Because the hemophiliac community is comparatively small, anyone active in it will know of at least a dozen relatives, friends, and acquaintances who have died as a result of this catastrophe.

But you do not have to be a hemophiliac to be affected by the contamination. Over time, it became apparent that hundreds more Canadians who had blood transfusions during surgery in the early 1980s were also infected. Some were given tainted blood during minor, elective operations that could have been postponed.

Hemophiliacs, who had to cope with their need for the blood's clotting factors all their lives, were the first to find out they had been contaminated with the virus that causes AIDS because of their frequent ties to the system. A regular pattern of clinic visits usually uncovered their HIV status. But transfused patients often were unaware of their incipient illness until they had an insurance test, or donated blood, or fell sick. In some cases, two parents have died, leaving orphaned children. Some of the ill are children, too young to have any notion of what was happening to them in those large, frightening institutions where the sick are cared for. Other victims didn't even know they had received transfused blood during their operations. Without that fundamental knowledge, they did nothing to protect their sexual partners from the deadly virus.

Many of those hundreds of people who were infected through transfusions have never been notified. Lax, frightened, litigation-shy, or hopelessly disorganized authorities did little or nothing to track them down. Bureaucrats and doctors debated whether the benefit of finding those who were stricken with a fatal virus was worth the cost. Now, ten to twelve years after the fact, they are urging people who were transfused during that period to be tested. While there's no cure for AIDS, many who found out years later could have been taking life-extending medication during that time. Some doctors, who should have known better, assumed the part best played by a deity and hid their knowledge about the HIV status of their patients. Politicians, approached for compensation because their agencies were involved, made secret deals and forced the fatally ill and their families to undertake costly legal actions. No one knows how many Canadians may have been indirectly infected or how many may have gone to their graves without knowing what killed them.

In May 1993, when a House of Commons sub-committee on health issues called for an inquiry into the events of the 1980s leading to the appalling tragedy, two members of Parliament, both physicians, urged anyone who had a blood transfusion between 1980 and 1985 to have a test done. Several provinces, including Ontario and Quebec, with the largest numbers of victims, followed up with announcements that they would test people who had received blood during that period. And new cases did show up. But it is almost certain that many more Canadians unknowingly continue to pass on the virus through sexual contact.

In June 1994, the Canadian Hospital Association finally issued a national recommendation that all persons who were blood-transfused between 1978 and 1985 be tested. The message is clear: don't wait for a personal invitation. Do it now!

The devastation of the Canadian hemophiliac community should concern all who depend on government and institutional bureaucracy to protect them from danger. In the case of the blood supply, the system was characterized by slow response to danger signals, a determination not to move from pre-established positions, and outright denial of the available evidence. True, the decision-makers of the day did not have all the information we have now. But there were both errors of commission and omission which could have been avoided. Government bureaucrats, the Red Cross, and other stakeholders failed those who relied upon the blood system for life. In some cases, viable alternatives were spurned or ignored for the pettiest of reasons. Mistakes were compounded by a refusal to follow up on the earlier failures. There were delays which put consumers of blood products at greater risk. Political exigencies, turf wars, and a stubborn rejection in some quarters of the notion that consumers might be right, or should even have a say in their treatment, all played a graphic role. Decisions were made that put safety second to budget trimming. Self-serving politicians pursued unachievable goals. Consumers — and in this book that means those who had these products injected into their bodies, not those who prescribe drugs — were self-destructively passive. Eyes were shut to mounting evidence, until it was too late. The Canadian system reacted slower and less decisively than in several other countries.

Today, Canada boasts one of the safest blood supplies in the world. But does the system react any better than it did in the 1980s? The events in Germany in the fall of 1993, when it was found that unscreened contaminated plasma passed through the system and infected people well after accurate screening was available, should give us pause. Some blood products derived from that tainted plasma did make their way to Canada and were used by patients. Fortunately, heat treatment had removed the danger. But once again, potentially dangerous blood, which should have been destroyed, slipped through the system. We are given assurances the blood supply is safer today than it has ever been, but would the chain of command cope better now if an as-yet unknown blood-borne virus arises? Perhaps. But old attitudes die hard. There are lessons still to be learned.

This book recounts the history of the events that led to the tragic infection of hundreds of Canadians. In its pages you will come across the names of many people whom the system failed — Justin Marche, Dr. Frank Terpstra, Bob Gibson, Eva Blaikie, and Stephen Christmas are only a few of them. The impact on the lives of those who depended on blood products will be examined. There will be a look at how the decision-makers in the system failed those they were supposed to protect. And some views will be offered on how the blood system can better serve the people it should serve — the Canadian public.

Chapter 1

CRUEL PARADOX

"We always say that our son died in 1992 but we lost him in 1989."
BILL MARCHE, 1993

At sixteen, Justin Marche changed from a mild-mannered, shy teenager into an unpredictable, obsessive young man seized by periods of violence and pyromania. This transformation shocked his parents, Rita and Bill, of Port au Port, Newfoundland.

Justin was a hemophiliac, suffering from a genetic blood disorder that was treated with clotting factors made from human blood. Those blood products, only available in recent decades, probably saved him from an early death. But, in a cruel paradox, they also stole his life.

There were many unanswered questions about acquired immuno-deficiency syndrome, better known as AIDS, when Justin became infected through the blood supply in the early 1980s. But much was known, too, and the victims of tainted blood say the authorities who had control over Canada's blood system could have made choices to halt or limit the damage.

Justin is one of at least a thousand Canadians — hemophiliacs and others who had blood transfusions — who became infected through the blood supply. It is now recommended that anyone who received blood products in the years 1979 to 1985 should have their blood tested for the virus believed to cause AIDS. There could still be hundreds of infected people who are unaware they have been damaged, either directly or indirectly through sexual contact with someone whose blood was contaminated.

For Justin, it is too late. After he had suffered a prolonged illness, characterized by severe AIDS dementia, the agony of Justin and his family terminated with his death in 1992. Or did it? The Marches, like many other victims of this tragedy, remain frustrated and bitter because governments and those who run the blood system have failed to recognize what happened to their lives.

Many who suffered through contamination of the blood supply feel that justice remains to be done. They believe, like the Marches, that the guardians of the system and those responsible for its operation must be forced to admit that errors were made, and that apologies and retribution are in order.

Rita Marche is angry that governments and authorities were slow to act even when it became apparent that the human immunodeficiency virus (HIV) was transmitted through blood. She and her husband, Bill, believe that if doctors had not held back information about the severity of Justin's illness, her only son might still be living.

"There were so many things that could have been done to prevent it that weren't done," Rita says. "I think that's what makes me so bitter. It didn't have to happen. They could have taken proper precautions."

Rita knew all about hemophilia. Her mother had two brothers who died very young, in the days before clotting factors were available. She also had two hemophiliac brothers who were infected by contaminated blood. One brother, Robert, died in April 1994, and the second is still living but has AIDS.

The bleeding disease was a fact of life for her, but AIDS was something else. "Until Justin was twelve years old, he lived a pretty normal life. We were so glad when concentrated blood-clotting factor came on the scene. It gave him a chance to do a lot of things that he probably wouldn't have been able to do otherwise. We thought it was great. We didn't realize that the same thing we thought was so great was going to take his life away.

"It has really devastated our family. Something that affects one affects all of them, because they know they're coming behind. It's scary for you because you know you've lost your son, but you're going to lose your brothers, too."

Justin's mental stability was completely thrown out of whack by his HIV infection. He would have violent rages during which Bill had to wrestle him to the floor. He threatened Rita. One bizarre manifestation was that he became obsessed with hair and would shave his head or even clip the family dog. Some days, he would forget how to eat or how to tie his shoelaces.

"He never returned to the person he was," explains Rita. "There were times when he was very violent and there were times when he was like a little three-year-old, wanting to hug you and to be kissed all the time. That wasn't like him either."

The most difficult to take, perhaps, was the fear and apprehension that came when Justin developed a fascination with fire. It led to trouble with the law and concern that the youth, then sixteen, would endanger the family's safety as well as his own.

"I got called at work by my brother-in-law," recalls Bill. "He said I should get home right away. When I got there, Justin wasn't in the house. I found him in the shed and there were burn spots on the floor, so I asked him what he was doing. He told me his professor had said that if you put enough gas on a fire you could actually extinguish it. I said maybe that's so, but it's not a very good experiment to try."

Bill and Rita were worried. They spent their days at work and Justin was home by himself. Rita's sister came over to work around the house and keep an eye on the lad. But worse was yet to come. One Sunday, on their daughter Carrie's thirteenth birthday, Justin, himself sixteen, banged on their bedroom door not long after midnight talking excitedly about a fire.

"He was saying, 'Dad, come and see the fire down on the wharf,'" Bill remembers. "He was just fascinated, really excited. I got up and, sure enough, a bunch of fishing buildings used during the summer months were blazing. Justin was laughing. The first thing that came to my mind was this must be his work, because I had heard him going out earlier.

"We went down and watched it. There was a thousand-gallon tank of gas, and he was waiting for it to burst, like in those TV shows. The next morning he was fresh as anything and laughing. It seemed unnatural. There was nothing funny going on. Someone had lost their property, and he was saying the police were stupid."

Later, Bill wandered down towards the site of the fire, still cordoned off, and he noticed in the grassy bank just behind his house five or six spots where fires had been set. He saw tracks in the sand and remembered Justin's sandy sneakers. Bill spotted a Mountie he knew at the fire site and explained to him about his suspicions and Justin's dementia.

"They had tracking dogs. That was all I wanted — them coming to the house with their dogs, getting Justin all scared. So the policeman came to the house and arrested Justin. We talked to the policeman afterwards and he said, 'I've seen a lot of hardened criminals, but I've never seen anyone like him. Calm, cool!' He said to Justin, 'I know you set the fire.' And Justin said, 'You have your opinion and I have mine, and I guess we'll have to let the judge decide.' This was a kid who four or five years earlier had thrown snowballs into the middle of the road, and when the police told him he shouldn't be doing that, he ran home and it took us an hour to get him to stop crying and tell us the awful thing he had done. He had been terrified of the police, yet here he was a hardened criminal who didn't show any remorse."

Hemophilia, the disorder that had wreaked so much havoc in Rita Marche's family, strikes about one in every five thousand males. It is a genetic condition passed through the females in a family and generally only affects the males. The disease prevents normal clotting of blood. An injury need not be severe to start the bleeding. A minor twist of an ankle or a bump against a table are insignificant events to someone with normal levels of blood-clotting factor; any bleeding that starts is quickly controlled by the body. To a hemophiliac, that kind of incident can be the start of an excruciatingly painful episode. Blood seeps into the joints and corrodes the protective surface of the bones. The pressure forces the joints apart and the damaged area swells to double or triple its size. In cases of severe hemophilia, continued bleeding and corrosion will lead to crippling if the episodes are not treated in time. Many hemophiliacs aged twenty or more, who grew up before clotting concentrates were available, walk with a permanent limp. Some have had joints replaced.

Here's how the genetic connection works: the sex of an individual is determined by x and y chromosomes — males have an xy makeup and females are xx. If a hemophiliac man with a "defective" x chromosome and a normal y marries a woman who has no connection with hemophilia, he will contribute his y chromosome to his sons. None of his boys, then, will be hemophiliacs, nor will they transmit the condition to future generations. His daughters, however, will receive his x chromosome and will all carry the gene that causes hemophilia. These daughters are likely to mate with men with normal xy chromosomes. Some of their sons could be hemophiliacs and others unaffected. Likewise, only some of the daughters will be carriers of the gene causing hemophilia.

According to the theoretical model, in a family of four children with two males and two females, one son would be a hemophiliac and one daughter a carrier of the disease. The other son and daughter would not be directly affected, and their children would escape the condition. Naturally, the real world is not always like that. All the daughters in a family could be carriers and all the sons hemophiliac. Or none might be affected. But the odds are that in any extended family, you will find a random mix. In Canada, there are an estimated 2,500 hemophiliacs. The exact number is uncertain because many of those with less severe incidence prefer not to make themselves known and, indeed, may not need treatment. Many hemophiliacs, even mild cases, have faced job discrimination from employers who either fear the unknown or who believe working time will be lost because of the disease.

Nature throws another curve, of course. While most cases of hemophilia can be tracked through several generations, it's estimated that between 20 to 40 per cent of hemophilia occurs through genetic mutation. In theory, then, it could appear in any family without any historical precedent.

There are at least fourteen separate substances in the blood that can have an effect on blood coagulation, so there are evidently several varieties of hemophilia. In cases of injury, these factors work in a sequence, sometimes known as a cascade, to repair the damage. When one factor is missing, the domino process doesn't work the way nature intended. The common garden variety of hemophilia is sometimes known as classical or hemophilia A, in which the clotting protein in the blood referred to as Factor VIII is missing or greatly reduced. The second most common variety is called Factor IX deficiency, hemophilia B, or Christmas disease, named after Stephen, the son of Canadian actor Eric Christmas. Stephen, who played a major role in the Canadian Hemophilia Society in the late 1980s, died in his forties in 1993 from AIDS. A third type is von Willebrand's disease, which affects both males and females equally and combines low Factor VIII levels with another deficiency. The second missing link here is called von Willebrand's Factor, which is needed to help form a firm plug of platelets when blood vessels are damaged. Although one might think having two missing elements in the blood would be worse than lacking one, von Willebrand's disease is generally not as severe as classical hemophilia.

There are varying degrees of severity of these diseases. There are, for example, documented cases of hemophiliacs who did not know they were vulnerable until they were into their forties. Some discovered their disease when they had a tooth extracted and the bleeding wouldn't stop. Others have found out when they were involved in traffic accidents. One young man discovered he was a hemophiliac after he twisted his knee during a parachute jump. Richard Burton had mild hemophilia. Another hemophiliac made the U.S. Olympic hockey team in 1992. Whether the condition is severe or mild, however, internal bleeding into the vital organs, joints, or muscles is far more serious than external cuts or abrasions.

Hemophilia has no respect for race or class. The disorder once was referred to as the "royal disease" because it afflicted so many of Europe's royalty descended from Queen Victoria, who was a carrier. Victoria had nine children, four males and five females. Two of her daughters, Alice and Beatrice, were carriers; one son, Leopold, was a hemophiliac. Alice's children married into the Russian and German royal families, and Beatrice into Spanish royalty. The best-known case was that of the Russian Crown Prince Alexei, Alice's grandson. Some historians claim the preoccupation of the royal family with Alexei's debilitating condition during a period of unrest contributed greatly to the Russian Revolution. But that connection to nobility was pure coincidence. The disease could appear in anyone's family, either submerged for many years, or through genetic mutation.

Until the middle of this century, it was rare for hemophiliacs, at least those with severe deficiencies, to survive into their twenties. Early on, the sole treatment consisted of pressure packs or ice. The pain was agonizing as uncoagulated blood seeped into knee or elbow joints, pushing them out of shape. For those who suffered head injuries or damage to the internal organs, there was little that could be done, except wait and hope. Transfusions of whole blood or plasma helped in later years, and products made from pig's blood were experimented with. These infusions were risky, expensive, and not overly reliable.

In 1965, Judith Pool, a postgraduate student in the United States, noticed that crystals rich in Factor VIII were the last to melt when frozen plasma was thawed. Her observation caused a revolution in the treatment of hemophilia. It led to the production of "cryoprecipitate," a clotting-factor product with much less volume than plasma. A new era had dawned. The new product promised longer and easier lives for hemophiliacs but it had a drawback. Cryoprecipitate was cumbersome. It had to be kept frozen until just before use and then mixed with saline as a medium to help it travel from the plastic bags in which it was stored into the veins of the recipient.

Travelling hemophiliacs would carry foam packs filled with the frozen product and dry ice. That was not to mention the bags of saline and the intravenous rigs for the slow drip infusions. A new, improved product soon became available, however.

Once the breakthrough came with cryoprecipitate, researchers took the process a step further and, after pooling plasma from large numbers of donors, came up with dried, more purified, bottled concentrates, which were widely circulated in the early 1980s. The volume was much smaller and freezing was not required, but the technology was still not terribly sophisticated.

Still, the new product meant hemophiliacs could now travel anywhere in the world as long as they had their handy vials of concentrate with them. The discovery offered a new lifestyle to most of those who suffered from blood coagulation disorders. Moreover, hundreds of young men who once faced an early death could live virtually normal lives, take on jobs they never could have aspired to, study at university, undergo complex operations, get married, have children, and not have to fear bleeding episodes that could incapacitate them. They could even take their supplies to work and school and, if they felt a bleed starting, inject concentrates to stop the bleeding from getting worse. Naturally, hemophilia was still a force to be reckoned with. Some men had suffered joint damage, for example, and faced surgery. Now, such medical treatment offered few more risks than for the average person. For about a decade, hemophiliacs thrived.

Then, a new tragedy overtook them.

"We always say," Bill Marche explains, "that our son died in 1992 but we lost him in 1989.

"There were times when you'd hate to come home," he recalls. "I hated coming through that door because you just didn't know what — honest to God — what you were going to meet. For the longest time this was just the way it was, and you can imagine the tension and the stress."

Seemingly happy times would erupt into horror. Once Rita, with

Carrie and her boyfriend, visited Justin in hospital. The youngsters left the room, leaving Rita alone with her son.

"I was sitting with him and we had a search-a-word, but he didn't know what he was doing. I asked him about a magazine. Arnold Schwarzenegger was on it — that was Justin's hero. He started quoting all of these things about Arnold Schwarzenegger, how many times he was champion of this and that. All of a sudden he took the pen and started coming at me with it, and his eyes were just wild. I tried to screech but I couldn't. I don't know how I got out the door."

Justin was put on anti-psychotic drugs, which helped bring his violent episodes under control. Because Newfoundland is a province with limited facilities, the authorities were not sure what to do with him. At one time they put him in an Alzheimer's ward, which provoked a violent reaction. After the arson, Justin was jailed and then sent to a rehabilitation centre for young offenders. He was isolated in one wing of the building. He refused to submit to a strip search because he had already undergone one when he was locked up. To punish him, they took away his mattress.

Rita was enraged. "I said, 'You've got my child in there. He's sick — he's got AIDS and he's a hemophiliac. He shouldn't be sleeping on the floor.' The next day they had him out of there."

In his final days, Justin received good care at the psychiatric ward of the Western Memorial Hospital in Corner Brook. There was much apprehension at first, with the staff nervous about a patient with AIDS, not to mention AIDS dementia. But they became close. The attendants came to be the pallbearers at Justin's funeral after he died on January 17, 1992.

"The nursing supervisor told me afterwards that Justin taught them more than any seminars or anything they could have read in a book," says Rita. "The personal side, I guess."

"He had good care in the end," adds Bill. "But we had to struggle for so long. I don't think anyone should have to do that. You should not have to fight for something like that."

For Bill and Rita, Justin's agonizing death sometimes seems far away and other times feels like yesterday. Their son is still a part of their lives and always will be, says Rita. But others, including Bill's family, have trouble handling it.

"My family has an expression that I hate for someone who dies," says Bill. "They say 'poor Justin' because he's dead, right? But I don't try to get around it. If I have something to say about him, I just say it."

Bill works as a provincial parks officer. When summer students come in, they are sometimes warned by others not to mention Justin. But Bill encourages them to ask: "I don't mind talking about my son, I enjoy talking about him. If you have something to ask me, go ahead. I could probably teach you a lot. Which is good. It's good for me, too."

The Marches are only one of about a thousand Canadian families devastated by the tainting of Canada's blood supply in the 1980s. Not all of the victims were hemophiliacs — at least a quarter were patients who received transfusions during operations. And it is only now that we are coming to realize the full impact of another virus that was carried by the tainted blood — hepatitis C.

The toll on blood-transfused patients who are not hemophiliacs may be much higher than was imagined when a national inquiry into the issue began in early 1994. The federal Laboratory Centre for Disease Control (LCDC) reported in August 1994 that an estimated 1,148 Canadians had been infected with HIV through transfusions between 1978 and 1985. The two experts who prepared the estimates, Robert Remis and Robert Palmer, said that at a minimum the number would be 942 infections and the grisly toll could be as high as 1,441. More than half of those infected likely had died of non-AIDS causes by 1994, the report further suggested. Only 419 blood-transfusion infections had been reported to national surveillance centres. There could be as many as 245, but most likely about 100, blood-transfused persons who might still be unaware of their infections.

In the case of hepatitis C, a generally less serious infection that afflicts a minority of individuals severely, a decision was made in 1986 not to follow the American lead and use indicator testing. Instead, a lengthy study was commissioned. That delay probably meant that at least ten thousand other Canadians were infected with a preventable post-transfusion disease.

Just the financial cost of the HIV disaster is staggering, not to mention the mental anguish and physical suffering of the victims and their survivors. It may already have cost Canada $500 million, and the costs are still rising. Federal compensation of $120 million has largely been paid out and an assistance program by the provinces is estimated $500 million. Add costs of welfare, drugs, and hospitalization, plus the hidden cost of lost productivity, and $500 million is an easily attainable figure. The irony is that some decisions seem to have been made to save an almost insignificant amount of money.

Surveying the human and financial cost arising from the tainted blood tragedy, one leader of the hemophilia community remarked in the fall of 1994: "It is never cost-effective to let a virus into the blood system."

Who was in charge of the vital blood supply in the early 1980s? Who made the decisions to use infected blood? Who, if anyone, is to blame for the devastation of these families and the deaths of those who were contaminated? Does the system work any better today?

Chapter 2

MEDICAL BACKWATER

*"We are all part of the blood system, at one end or another,
and we can be at both ends. We can be donors at
one point and patients at the other."*

DR. ROSLYN HERST, MEDICAL DIRECTOR OF THE TORONTO RED CROSS,
FEBRUARY 1994

Although Canada's blood system has the reputation of being one of
the world's best, critics see it as a shapeless entity lacking accountability and without any one agency in charge. In times of peril, as in
the AIDS crisis of the 1980s, the system has been slow to react and
devoid of leadership. Justice Horace Krever, launching his multi-
million-dollar inquiry in the fall of 1993, reflected that it may not
even be a "system."

There are several key players, and many walk-on parts, in the
story. Some of the names have changed since the crisis of the mid-
1980s, but the structure is essentially the same. The central role,
happily accepting praise when all goes well and deflecting blame when
trouble erupts, belongs to the Canadian Red Cross Society. The Red
Cross is almost synonymous with blood collection and distribution
in this country, even though the agency engages in a wide range of
other activities from home services to swimming programs. Its goals
have been summed up as the improvement of health, the prevention
of disease, and the mitigation of suffering.

For many years, the society has been a powerful force in Canada's
medical system. Try to draw a chart of the blood system, and the Red
Cross is the common thread connecting the various parts. The role

of the donor recruitment side of the Red Cross is to attract, cajole, beg, guide, or shame prospective donors into taking the time to give blood at fixed or mobile clinics. Each year more than one million donations, in peak years considerably more, are collected in Canada.

Once the donor is through the door, the transfusion service takes his or her blood and may send it on to manufacturers, known as fractionators, to be processed into a variety of products, including clotting factors. Once processed, these are returned to the Red Cross and relayed to hundreds of hospitals and treatment centres. If a blood-clearing agency like the Red Cross did not exist, one would have to be created.

The Canadian Red Cross was incorporated in 1909. After the society acquired experience in the war years organizing blood transfusion services, the federal government asked that it set up a parallel civilian service. Two basic principles guided the voluntary Canadian blood system: donors were not paid for giving their blood, and recipients were not charged for receiving it. By the early 1980s, government money paid 100 per cent of technical costs for the blood transfusion service and 80 per cent of donor recruitment costs.

The national nature of the blood system is, in part at least, due to the Red Cross. Collection and distribution are done through seventeen regional centres and, as the House of Commons subcommittee on health issues pointed out in 1993, operated without heed to provincial boundaries. "Blood and blood products are freely exchanged between provinces; distribution, therefore, is on a national basis." The MPs noted that the blood system is unique among healthcare programs: "It is an essentially national system under the jurisdiction of the provinces and the territories, which provide all of the government funding."

Dr. Roger Perrault, national director of blood services for the Red Cross in the crucial period between 1974 and 1986, told the federal sub-committee in 1993 that there were essentially three parts to the system. Policy and funding were under the aegis of provincial governments; the operational arm was the Red Cross; and the third part was made up of the consumers — commonly identified as the doctors, the hospitals, and the end-using patients. "Whatever changes are going to be contemplated in the future, we will have to take those three arms into account," he said.

This tripartite system sounds as if it might offer a set of checks and balances. In truth, like a tribal shaman, the Red Cross has been the repository of the esoteric secrets of the blood-products universe. Not only does it run the collection and distribution systems, the Red Cross negotiates contracts with manufacturers and has kept those details to itself, sometimes even shutting out the government agency that foots the bill. It has produced a blood product, cryoprecipitate, which plays an important part in the story of tainted blood. Governments might pay the tab and try to regulate the system, physicians might prescribe the products to be used, and public-health authorities might watch for infections arising from the blood supply, but in times of stress all have deferred to the expertise and inside knowledge of the Red Cross.

Like many Canadian institutions under shared authority, the blood system has been at times in danger of paralysis. This was especially true during the crisis of the early 1980s when blood authorities, before they would consider taking action, required scientific proof that was unobtainable at the time. A response was demanded and, instead, confusion abounded. The question arose: who's in charge here?

Before the AIDS epidemic arrived, in the late 1970s, a number of threats to the smooth functioning of the blood system were surfacing. A report to the federal and provincial ministers of health in 1979 said the Canadian blood and blood product system was unstable and untenable, and required "long-term policy commitments" by the two levels of government.

There was a trend towards increased reliance on foreign-owned fractionators of blood, the report said. The Red Cross and Canada's main manufacturer of blood products, Connaught Laboratories of Toronto, had developed a "continuing unstable and antagonistic relationship." Connaught had been taken over in the early 1970s by the Canada Development Corporation. The federal government was the

CDC's largest shareholder. Ottawa hoped to entice shareholders from the general public and demanded a better bottom line from the company. It was around that time that Connaught began making noises about commercial blood collections, through which donors would be paid for their plasma. The Red Cross and others, notably hemophiliacs, viewed this possibility with alarm, saying it would undermine the volunteer donor system, which was regarded with pride in Canada. Canadians had always boasted of having a far superior and less risky system than existed in the United States, where some blood was obtained from volunteers and the rest from commercial operations. The common perception was that the payment of donors attracted drunks and drug addicts who would do anything for a bottle or a fix, or prostitutes and others who might transmit disease through blood.

One senior medical officer, testifying in March 1994 before the Krever inquiry, said that as a general rule, payment for blood increases the danger of transfusion reactions. "The more you pay for blood, the greater incentive there is to misrepresent its quality."

In the late 1970s and early 1980s, debate over the structure of Canada's blood system led to the creation of a federal-provincial Ad Hoc Committee on Plasma Fractionation. That committee recommended early in the 1980s the establishment of a Canadian Blood Authority to "maintain, monitor, develop, and direct" the system. The proposed authority could respond to social and technological change, it said, while maintaining the principles of the blood system.

As often happens, one bureaucratic institution gave birth to another, and in the summer of 1981, a second ad hoc committee reaffirmed the principles that had guided the blood system. There were four guidelines:

- To protect the system by promoting opportunities for Canadians to voluntarily donate blood for society's general benefit, and by responsibly managing the resource

- To ensure Canadian self-sufficiency of blood products by reducing dependence upon foreign sources, especially purchased plasma
- To ensure that blood products are available to those who need them by reinforcing the tradition that no payment is made for blood or plasma and no charge is levied on it
- To maintain the non-profit status of the blood system; any charge more than the real cost of producing a blood fractionation product would be considered profit

The call for a blood authority was endorsed by health ministers, but when the creature was born in 1981 it was named the Canadian Blood Committee, or CBC. On it sat a representative of each of the provinces and the federal government. The secretariat was headed by an executive director from the federal Health Department, and staff were also federal employees. But the CBC had no legislative authority and no public accountability. It was never incorporated, and had no power to contract or borrow money.

The CBC was to direct the system according to principles set out by the health ministers. It would review and approve programs and budgets of the Red Cross blood donor and transfusion services, "subject to the concurrence of the provinces and territories." A central goal was to formulate a national blood policy, but such a policy did not emerge from the hours of discussion and the reams of paperwork.

In the aftermath of the AIDS crisis in 1991, the provinces and territories got together and incorporated a new structure to replace the CBC. Known as the Canadian Blood Agency (CBA), its objective is to "direct, coordinate, and finance the various elements of the Canadian blood system requiring national direction." The federal government is not part of the new agency. Unlike its predecessor, the CBA has been given authority by the provinces to make contracts and borrow funds as deemed necessary. The agency's executive director has a line of credit that allows the borrowing of up to $3.5 million if required.

Since the hiring of the executive director, William Dobson, in October 1991, the CBA has been flexing its muscles, largely to the dismay and at the expense of the Red Cross. Dobson told the Krever inquiry in February 1994 that his preference is to use "persuasion, appeals to the greatest good, and selling a deal on its merits." But the Agency has trod on Red Cross toes by trimming budgets unilaterally. Through the full exercise of its power, the Agency could also spell trouble for consumers of blood products. "We have an interest in getting our consumption levels down, not just because of the cost, but because it's safer," Dobson said.

The federal government plays a vital role in the system through the Bureau of Biologics, a division of the Health Protection Branch that regulates blood and blood products, as well as other pharmaceuticals produced from humans or animals. These products are regarded as biological drugs under the Food and Drugs Act. The bureau's self-described responsibility "is to ensure safe and efficacious biological drugs are available to the Canadian public, which is accomplished through licensing, inspection and lot by lot approvals." Testing and evaluation are done on new drugs and manufacturing sites are inspected. Since 1989, bureau officials conduct regular inspections of Red Cross blood collection centres before licences are renewed. In some instances, either because of staff shortages or lack of expertise, there has been slippage.

A tough regulatory regime is required to protect Canadians from health hazards. Nowhere is this more true than in the case of biological drugs. With chemically produced drugs, the results are consistent and predictable. Biologicals, a federal official told the Krever inquiry in 1994, are more complex. Things can go wrong along the way.

"You just can't assume that a batch produced one day is going to be the same in terms of potency or purity or sensitivity or whatever as the batch produced the next day," said Dann Michols, executive director of Health Canada's drugs directorate. "Consequently, more can go wrong, and we need to ensure that each batch is equal to the standards that we have approved." Thus, each time a manufacturer produces the drug, it must send samples to be tested.

If emergencies occur, the Health Protection Branch, of which the Bureau of Biologics is a part, would be notified and federal officials would have control over the manufacturer, the Red Cross, and the clinics distributing the offending product. Each of those must have emergency procedures in place to get a licence. "And they would have to ensure the procedures work to keep their licence," Michols said.

Another group of players are the so-called fractionators — manufacturers that take whole blood or plasma and break it down into a variety of products which can be used to treat a wide range of conditions and maladies. Connaught was the only Canadian fractionator of significance, producing blood-clotting concentrates in the 1980s before it dropped out. (Two other Canadian firms, one in Montreal and one in Winnipeg, never achieved any meaningful production of concentrates.)

The other key fractionators are all U.S.-based. Most important of these to Canada is Cutter Laboratories, part of Miles Inc., which produces coagulants from Canadian volunteer plasma and then ships them back to this country. But because of production difficulties at Connaught and insufficient Canadian plasma supply to Cutter, other "commercial" concentrates made from U.S.–source blood were purchased to supplement the Canadian supply. Cutter supplied some and so did other producers such as Armour, Baxter-Hyland, and Alpha. A small amount of concentrates was also purchased from European firms, especially Immuno of Austria. The commercial products bought from the United States are believed by many to have been the initial source of HIV infection in Canada.

Once these blood products were purchased by the Red Cross, they were turned over to Blood Transfusion Service regional centres and moved on to hospital blood banks, hemophilia specialty clinics in major cities, or in rare cases directly to hemophiliacs. Doctors specializing in hemophilia, sometimes in consultation with the patient, prescribed or administered the clotting factors. As the AIDS crisis developed among the blood-transfused, both the Red Cross and the

Bureau of Biologics hastened to say the choice of a specific drug was a matter between the treaters and the treated. It wasn't their job.

The volunteer organization representing hemophiliacs in Canada is the Canadian Hemophilia Society (CHS). Although it claims to represent everyone with the disease, whether they carry a membership card or not, it has often struggled to develop and maintain a steady and supportive volunteer base. Many hemophiliacs, until they run into trouble, have tended to be apathetic and complacent, preferring to ignore their disease. Living a "normal" life and not being set apart from others in society has generally been very important to them. Indeed, many show few signs of their condition and prefer to pass through life without drawing attention to it. For mild and even moderate cases, this can often be accomplished with today's medical knowledge.

The society is divided into provincial chapters, which not infrequently are at odds with the national organization. The picture is even more complex in Ontario, where there have been up to six regions with varying degrees of strength, often engaged in their own spats with the provincial board.

Over the years, the CHS has struggled — with varying degrees of success — to have its voice heard in corporate and government boardrooms. Society officials believe that as representatives of the prime users of blood products, they should be part of the policy-making process. But even today, the Red Cross does not have a single blood-consumer representative on its board.

Blood users have paid a heavy price for this refusal by the authorities to treat them as partners. "On many occasions, when the CHS brought forward very serious concerns about the safety of the products, they were passed around the circuit of the Canadian Blood Committee, the Bureau of Biologics, and Red Cross," the CHS complained in a brief to the federal government in 1988. "There was no national strategy for preventing the transmission of HIV through the Canadian blood system."

Another key player in the story is the society's Medical and Scientific Advisory Committee (MSAC), which chiefly comprises blood specialists and other treaters of hemophiliac patients and which provides counsel to the volunteer group. At crucial times in the mid-1980s, the MSAC appeared directionless and paralyzed. One observer of the scene reflects today that despite its title, the MSAC spent most of its sessions debating economics and politics.

In 1983, when drawing up a "communications chain" for recall of suspected contaminated blood products, Dr. Roslyn Herst, a Red Cross centre medical director, identified key players from source to end user. They were the fractionators, the national Red Cross Blood Transfusion Centre, the regional blood transfusion centres, hospital blood banks and blood-bank doctors, treating physicians, recipients of products, and the national and provincial sections of the Canadian Hemophilia Society. "In order to make blood transfusion as safe as possible, close communication and cooperation are required between the various professional groups involved in the chain from blood donor to patient," she wrote.

But it was a complex chain. If one link failed, there could be trouble, serious trouble.

Today, the Red Cross national office occupies a palatial red-brick building with grey-green trim, complete with courtyard and fountain, perched on a hill above Ottawa's Rideau River. In spring, the suburban air is sweet with the smell of crabapple and honeysuckle blossoms.

Stephen Vick, a veteran of eighteen years with the Red Cross and now assistant national director of manufacturing, describes the new Red Cross as a corporate entity concerned with good pharmaceutical manufacturing processes and quality. Before the AIDS tragedy, he says, transfusion services were "a backwater of medicine and we were considered almost an adjunct of the hospital blood banks." There has been a major cultural change worldwide in the business, a change which has stemmed from the disaster of the 1980s.

What was the state of the Canadian Red Cross a decade ago?

Those devoted volunteers who had given so much personal effort to its worthy causes might have been surprised if they had known of the inner turmoil of the mid- to late-1980s.

Regional medical directors were frustrated at the apparent reluctance of the national office to move more swiftly against the danger to the blood supply. The phrase frequently repeated was that the Red Cross, like the church, was "not a democracy." Many senior, well-qualified people left the agency at the time.

Dr. Gail Rock, a former Red Cross medical director and researcher who was fired in 1988, sums up the feelings many former employees had towards the Red Cross. There is a reliable blood program in spite of the system, not because of it, Rock told authors of an article that appeared in the *Canadian Medical Association Journal* in 1990. "We have essentially given a monopoly on blood transfusion in the country to what is essentially a non-medical organization," she told the parliamentary sub-committee on health issues early in 1993. She called it an organization that ignored advice from its medical directors and resisted suggestions that AIDS could be transmitted through the blood. That was costly for those who depended upon the system for life.

The article by Peter Morgan and Lynne Cohen described the Red Cross as a "heavily centralized hierarchy," which over the years had "dismissed, discouraged, or antagonized several well-respected professionals." One example of management problems was the delay in screening of blood for HIV.

Among others who left the Red Cross in the mid-1980s was Joan Kent, former Ontario director of blood donor recruitment. "My perception of the Red Cross blood program in Ontario from 1982 to 1986 is that it was a bumbling, self-serving system controlled for the most part by volunteers and staff who spent most of their time infighting and manoeuvring for power," she told the parliamentary sub-committee.

Red Cross bureaucrats certainly saw their role as the traditional guardians of the blood system, which gave them special rights. When a draft national blood policy was put together in 1987 after the well-documented HIV contamination of the blood supply, the Red Cross wanted first dibs. Roger Perrault wrote Denise Leclerc-Lecavalier, then executive director of the Canadian Blood Committee. "We hope our comments will be taken into consideration before circulation to the other agencies," he said. This showed remarkable chutzpah, considering that Red Cross sluggishness had been a major contributor to the dissemination of tainted blood two years earlier.

There's another way of looking at the system. "Each and every day a volunteer donor comes into the clinic and donates because he or she believes they are going to help someone," Dr. Tom Bowen of Calgary told the Krever inquiry. A former medical director who quit in 1985 after becoming frustrated with the bureaucracy of the system, Bowen praised the grassroots volunteer component.

"Those clinics were successful because the volunteers worked their butts off to make the clinic organized and to get the donor population in. I think the system works best as a grassroots-based organization where they think they are helping their own community."

In truth, the blood system depends on volunteer donors who want to help save lives. At the other end are the recipients, people like Justin Marche, who need the blood that is freely given. All the bureaucracy in between is intended to help the exchange network function. In the 1980s the gears of this elaborate machinery seized and the system failed to protect the public.

Chapter 3

CLIPPED WINGS

"Hemophiliacs serve as an early warning system for the safety of the blood supply. We were a blinking yellow warning about the blood supply, and we didn't want the industry to wait for the red light to take action."

ALAN BROWNSTEIN, DIRECTOR OF THE U.S. NATIONAL
HEMOPHILIA FOUNDATION, IN EARLY 1983

Ken Poyser was exultant in the spring of 1981 when he took over as president of the Canadian Hemophilia Society. He was, after all, the first hemophiliac to head the organization since Frank Schnabel of Montreal founded the society in 1953. Poyser, a young Albertan accountant, had ended the procession of parents and sympathetic friends who had led the CHS for nearly three decades.

To an outsider, it might seem odd that Poyser was so upbeat in his first annual report to the society, and that he made such a point of noting that five of the seven members of the national executive were hemophiliacs. A reader oblivious to the toll the disease exacted on the young might expect a hemophilia society to be led by a hemophiliac. But Poyser's election was proof that young hemophiliacs, with the help of new blood-clotting agents, were now surviving into adulthood and taking control of their lives.

"I have lived!" Poyser wrote joyfully. "Lived agonizingly through the years without treatment, suffered through the years of plasma, painfully carried on through the years of cryoprecipitate, and experienced the privilege of being alive in the age of concentrate. I know the pain of hemophilia."

These were, indeed, happy times for those who had to cope with hemophilia. A parent with a child born with the crippling disease in 1981 could legitimately expect the infant to live a normal life span. Specialist clinics were being set up in most of Canada's major cities, providing physiotherapy, social support, and dental work, as well as the doctoring needed. Research continued on new blood-clotting products, and there was even talk of a future in which artificially produced agents would be available, skirting the perils of infection inherent in blood extracted from humans. Except in traumatic circumstances and for a minority who had inhibitors that prevented the full effectiveness of infused blood products, the disorder seemed destined to be a mere annoyance for most Canadian hemophiliacs.

"Hemophiliacs can now enjoy an active life," Poyser reported. "Hemophilic children can run and jump; they can laugh and play without the horrible fear of impending pain. Hemophilic youths can more easily intermingle with other youths without the fears of being different or without the unfortunate glare of society attached to those who limp or suffer from physical impairment. Hemophilic adults, probably crippled but who have survived the 'put-ice-on-it ages' can rejoice with their new-found freedom. This is the freedom of independence: to rely no longer on doctors or hospitals, parents or society, but rather to participate actively in society with a career, a spouse, a family."

Over the next decade and more, this bright vision of the future was destroyed for many hemophiliacs.

One cause of Poyser's optimism was the introduction of a breed of superior blood-clotting products. In 1979, the first vial of dried Factor VIII clotting concentrate was produced and delivered from Canadian-donated blood. Earlier, factor made from U.S. blood had been imported, but its use was just becoming widespread. The dried concentrates made life much easier for hemophiliacs. Their movements were virtually limitless now. The new products were compact, portable, and didn't require freezing. They were also much more potent in stopping bleeds.

Human blood has been likened to a river that flows through many courses throughout the body and is the habitat for an astonishing variety of living cells. About half of the blood consists of numerous red blood cells which carry oxygen, less prominent white cells which fight disease, and platelets which help blood clot in times of injury. The other half is known as plasma, which contains a wide range of proteins, minerals, fats, and the like. Plasma can be separated into blood derivatives and used to treat a range of illnesses. Among the products that can be separated from plasma are Factor VIII and Factor IX, used by hemophiliacs to halt or control their bleeding.

The "active ingredient" in Factor VIII blood products is called antihemophilic factor and is measured in International Units. One unit measures the amount of Factor VIII found in one millilitre of fresh human plasma. Judith Pool's discovery of enriched Factor VIII in cryoprecipitate represented a ten-fold improvement. When low-purity dried concentrates arrived, they were another great step ahead. Today's high-purity products have 50 to 150 times more Factor VIII as the same volume of fresh plasma, and the new "ultra" high-purity ones are between 2,000 and 5,000 units a milligram — so high that to be infused, stable human albumin, another blood product, must be added.

Ken Poyser would not have known when he wrote his upbeat message to hemophiliacs in 1981 that a mysterious new disease was appearing among gay Americans in the Los Angeles area. The *Morbidity and Mortality Weekly*, compelling reading for those concerned with emerging fatal conditions, reported in June that five men had been admitted to three different hospitals with an unusual form of pneumonia caused by a low form of animal life known as the *Pneumocystis carinii* protozoan. Although the protozoan is not uncommon, it is generally not a danger to healthy humans. The pneumonia usually appeared only in infants or in people with severely damaged immune systems. That summer, cases of a rare cancer known as Kaposi's sarcoma also showed up in young men in New York.

The Centers for Disease Control in Atlanta had determined at the end of August 1981 that there were 110 exceptional cases with these rare diseases in the United States. They were all male and homosexual. They also had severely impaired immune systems. Early on, the disease was known as GRID (gay-related immune deficiency). Soon, however, it became apparent the disease could be acquired by others, including intravenous drug users and people who had received blood or blood derivatives. A year after the first cases, the Centers for Disease Control said heterosexual drug users of both sexes accounted for one of every five patients. A clamour grew for the renaming of the disease and an end to the view that the disease was exclusive to homosexuals. It was renamed acquired immunodeficiency syndrome, or AIDS.

AIDS is caused by one of a class of viruses known as retroviruses that contain the enzyme reverse transcriptase. When the retrovirus enters the human body, it selectively infects the T-cell lymphocytes, which play a major role in protecting the body against unwanted intruders. The virus invades the cell and once inside uses the reverse transcriptase to incorporate itself into the DNA of the human cells. When it is time to replicate, the invaded cell creates more viruses and these are released to spread throughout the body.

"Literally, it's hijacking a human cell," Dr. Alexander Klein of Toronto told Justice Horace Krever's blood inquiry early in 1994. Once the hijacking is done, it is difficult to target the retrovirus because it's not possible for the body's immunity defenders to distinguish infected cells from normal ones. Tests for HIV have focused on the antibodies the body produces to fight off the infection, rather than on the virus itself, because the virus hides away in apparently normal cells.

Perhaps a third of HIV-infected people experience a short flu-like illness soon after contact with the virus. But because their immune systems are healthy then, they readily fight off the infection. It is not until the T-cell (or CD-4) count drops below 200 cells per cubic millimetre of blood that the weakened body becomes exposed to a wide range of opportunistic infections. (A normal range is between 400 to 1,000.) These infections are the killers, not AIDS itself.

It's now believed that HIV transmission through blood or its derivatives is the most "efficient" way for the virus to spread, with a chance of infection greater than 90 per cent for a single exposure. The risk of transfer of virus from infected mother to unborn child is estimated at 30 per cent. The rate of infection through sex — although accounting for the vast majority of AIDS cases — is considerably lower, about 1 per cent chance per single exposure. Naturally, in the case of sexual transmission the risk is heightened because of the frequency of exposures.

With the number of cases mounting in the United States, it seemed inevitable that the disease would appear in Canada. In February 1982, eight months after the earliest reports, the first case was described in this country. With the focus on the gay community, AIDS was not regarded as a threat by hemophiliacs or other users of blood. When an occasional clairvoyant raised the possibility that AIDS might be transmitted through blood, they were accused by doctors, blood authorities, and some hemophiliacs of being alarmist. But soon there was evidence that blood products were a source of danger.

In July 1982, a month after the Centers for Disease Control reported that intravenous drug users were being infected, the first three cases among hemophiliacs were publicly confirmed in widespread locations in the United States. One twenty-seven-year-old Ohio man fell ill in July 1981 and died two months after the CDC announced its findings, following *Pneumocystis carinii* pneumonia (PCP). Being gay, it was now clear, was not a prerequisite for AIDS.

The U.S. Public Health Service moved quickly and invited government health officials and regulators, blood-bank representatives, and leaders of the National Hemophilia Foundation (the U.S. equivalent of the Canadian Hemophilia Society) and of the National Gay Task Force to a meeting on July 27, 1982. "The possibility exists that [AIDS] is occurring in patients with hemophilia," a summary of the meeting says. "If the PCP observed in three patients with hemophilia represents the same process as seen in other groups with AIDS, then a possible mode of transmission is via blood products, in this case

Factor VIII concentrate." Hemophiliacs used large amounts of Factor VIII each year and were potentially exposed to material pooled from thousands of blood donors. An "active surveillance system" should be set up to watch for other suspicious cases in hemophiliacs.

One of the early American cases was reported by Dr. Man-Chiu Poon, later prominent in Canada's hemophilia community. Poon and his colleagues wrote of a fifty-five-year-old man with no other supposed risk factors — he was not gay, not a drug user — who had been hospitalized and developed pneumonia.

The appearance of the syndrome in hemophiliacs was significant. Whatever caused the disease survived the filtration process used to remove impurities in the production of blood-clotting concentrates. The culprit had to be extremely small. Some scientists concluded a virus was implicated.

Early in 1983, news arrived from France that a virus called lymphadenopathy-associated virus, or LAV, had been isolated. Lymphadenopathy means disease of the lymph nodes, which supply a variety of white corpuscles known as lymphocytes to the blood and remove bacteria and foreign particles from bodily fluids. (Later American research identified a virus known as HTLV-III. Both were eventually accepted as the human immunodeficiency virus or HIV.)

More American studies reported a "striking reduction" in the T-lymphocyte cells of hemophiliacs, abnormalities similar to those found in homosexual men critically ill with PCP. Caution was being advised in the use of clotting-factor concentrates. North Carolina specialists Gilbert White and Henry Lesesne correctly predicted the forthcoming disaster. Although the incidence of AIDS among hemophiliacs was low, they wrote, the series of patients with T-cell abnormalities who were not yet showing opportunistic infections "suggests we may be seeing the tip of the iceberg."

They qualified these remarks by saying the changes do not necessarily indicate immune deficiency. Then they raised the dilemma: how should physicians treat hemophiliacs, knowing that an infusion of concentrates may cause AIDS and that withholding them may result in uncontrolled bleeding? It is a question that resounds to this day.

Other studies indicated patients treated with cryoprecipitate had normal cell counts compared with those treated with concentrates. White and Lesesne explained how they were going to cope: they would cancel elective procedures, reduce doses, and switch some patients from concentrate to cryoprecipitate. "But these are only stopgap measures for what may be a major health hazard in this and other patient populations."

Some Canadian authorities had quickly spotted the potential danger. In August 1982, the federal Bureau of Biologics of the Health Protection Branch asked the Red Cross to alert doctors to watch for hemophiliacs with AIDS and to coordinate laboratory studies. "There is a theoretical risk that an unknown transmissible agent present in AHF (anti-hemophilic factor) products may be responsible for AIDS in these patients," its briefing notes said. The Bureau did not act to remove or control the presumed offending product, nor did it propose alternatives. Rather than continuing an active and interventionist role to protect and monitor the blood supply, the Bureau dropped out of sight for two years. The August 1982 intervention was the only time the Bureau clearly acted with commendable speed.

Doctors, Red Cross officials, and public health authorities met in Toronto on December 2, 1982, to thrash out a project that would study AIDS in volunteer groups of gays and hemophiliacs. If American reports were true that intravenous blood products were a route of AIDS transmission, it would have "serious and far-reaching implications with respect to donation and distribution of blood products," says a summary of the meeting.

In January 1983, medical directors of the Canadian Red Cross discussed a report by a working group on immunology and virology that suggested AIDS could be transmitted through blood. The view was becoming widely accepted. Although conclusive evidence was lacking, it was suggested that "reasonable" attempts should be made to limit blood donations from groups with an "unacceptably high risk" of AIDS.

The evidence of infection through concentrates was grimly piling

up. But there were powerful corporate naysayers — those who prof-
ited from the blood industry. Frustration with the reluctance to accept
the accumulating knowledge led to the celebrated outburst on January
4, 1983, by Don Francis of the Centers for Disease Control. American blood bankers had been reluctant at a CDC-sponsored conference
in Atlanta to accept the notion of AIDS transmission through blood.
Francis demanded to know the threshold of deaths required before
the idea would be taken seriously.

The meeting was a wild and woolly affair. John Hink, a Cutter
Laboratories representative, reported in a company memo that the
objective had been to arrive at meaningful recommendations for
action. "However, difficulties in communication and political power
struggles made progress towards these objectives difficult. The
anti-discrimination position of the gays, self-serving comments of
blood bankers, and lack of data to provide legitimacy to many proposals resulted in an overall stalemate."

Two days after the Atlanta meeting, Francis issued a memoran-
dum calling for deferral of donors who were drug users, sexually
promiscuous (either heterosexual or homosexual), those who had
sexual contacts with either of those groups, anyone who had lived
in Haiti in the previous five years, or who had a positive test for
hepatitis B antibodies. These deferrals, Francis suggested, would
eliminate over three-quarters of infected donors and defer about
5 per cent of American donors. It would also add a five-dollar additional cost to each donation of blood and plasma. "These seem to
be small prices for preventing a serious disease and a potentially
dangerous panic.

"For hemophiliacs, I fear it might be too late," he added. Francis
said if cell ratio data collected thus far "was reflective of pre-AIDS, a
third to half of all hemophiliacs might already be exposed. Despite
this grim picture among hemophiliacs, however, we should do our
utmost to prevent further exposure and recommendations for plasma
products should be made." He foresaw that the virus could spread to
other users of blood products.

Bruce Evatt, a colleague of Don Francis's, was worried, too. He had written as far back as July 1982 that hemophiliacs "would be prime candidates to develop this syndrome." At a March 1983 meeting of the American Blood Resources Association in Las Vegas, Evatt said he was convinced there was much more infection than had been reported. "About half the hemophilic population perceived to have abnormal T-cell function can be expected to come down with AIDS." reported Hink in an internal Cutter memo on Evatt's talk. Unfortunately, Evatt and Francis proved to be excellent forecasters. And like many other prophets, they were largely ignored.

Some U.S. blood bankers, at least, felt the Centers for Disease Control was engaged in self-promotional games. An American Red Cross memo from February 1983 agreed that there was strong evidence that AIDS was transmissible through Factor VIII concentrates. But it noted that the CDC cannot be relied on to provide "scientific, objective, unbiased leadership."

"Even if the evolving evidence of an epidemic wanes, CDC is likely to play up AIDS — it has long been noted that CDC increasingly needs a major epidemic to justify its existence," the memo said. By "playing up" AIDS, the CDC was able to dodge funding cuts ordered by Ronald Reagan's administration and get $15 million for a new virology lab, the memo continued. "To the extent the industry (American Red Cross, Council of Community Blood Centers, American Association of Blood Banks) sticks together against CDC, it will appear to some segments of the public at least that we have a self-interest which is in conflict with the public interest, unless we can clearly demonstrate that CDC is wrong."

As quarrels continued, some hemophilia specialists were mulling over ways of avoiding the catastrophe that would likely arise from contaminated blood. In mid-January 1983, the National Hemophilia Foundation held a strategy meeting attended by manufacturers and blood bankers. Three Canadians were there: Dr. John Derrick, a senior officer of the Canadian Red Cross; Dr. Hanna Strawczynski, then chairing the medical advisors to the Canadian Hemophilia Society; and her Montreal colleague, Dr. Christos Tsoukas, an immunologist at Montreal General Hospital.

The meeting produced recommendations for the use of alternatives to dried concentrates: expanded use of cryoprecipitate, pooled from smaller numbers of donors than the concentrates or even produced from single donors, was one possibility; the use of desmopression or DDAVP, often employed by mild hemophiliacs or those with von Willebrand's disease to unlock the body's own clotting capacity; the use of freeze-dried concentrates derived from smaller donor pools; cutbacks in the amount and frequency of use; and the exclusion of blood donors from high-risk groups.

Three weeks later, Strawczynski met medical advisors to the Canadian Hemophilia Society. Similar recommendations to those adopted by the NHF were drafted. In messages to hemophiliacs, however, the threat was downplayed. "The risk for a patient with hemophilia of coming down with this disease is minimal at this time," Strawczynski wrote in *Hemophilia Today*, the CHS newsletter. "The experts from the Centers for Disease Control do not recommend any change in the use of blood products; consequently, it is not advised to change in any way the infusion treatment of hemophilia."

A somewhat different message, revealing greater concern, was being distributed to physicians who treated hemophiliacs. The draft sent by Strawczynski on February 17, 1983, suggested the use of cryoprecipitate for hemophiliacs who had never before used dried concentrates. Cryoprecipitate users who had to travel or could not get their preferred product should use concentrates made from plasma collected from Canadian donors. Newly diagnosed or mild Factor IX hemophiliacs should use fresh-frozen plasma whenever possible. Other patients were to continue using concentrates but to treat bleeds early, or to revert to the old days and use splints to immobilize limbs. The idea was to avoid large doses and prolonged treatment. Postponement of all elective surgery was urged until more information was available about the transmission of AIDS.

Strawczynski also called for "serious efforts" to exclude blood donors who might transmit AIDS. This could include an "educational campaign" to discourage high-risk groups, specifically male homosexuals and Haitian immigrants, from donating. The Red Cross should use specific questions in a donor questionnaire to detect symptoms of AIDS, including swollen lymph nodes, night sweats, weight loss, and unexplained fever, she said.

Meanwhile, steps should be taken to increase the supply and provide for the "most rational distribution" of cryoprecipitate. Strawczynski also recommended urgent steps to make Canada self-sufficient in volunteer donor plasma and fractionated products.

Clearly, there was considerable concern about the status of the blood supply, and even if the guilty virus had not yet been identified, these steps would have gone a long way to protecting consumers.

Don Francis's co-workers at the Centers for Disease Control — Evatt, James Curran, and Dale Lawrence — were busy spelling out why tainted blood could pose a severe risk to hemophiliacs and were adding a new group: surgery patients who required transfusions. Each lot of clotting factor, they noted in an article in the *Annals of Internal Medicine,* was produced from 2,500 to 22,500 individual donations. About 800 lots a year were produced in the United States, each containing about 500,000 units. The average hemophiliac infused 30,000 to 50,000 units a year.

This meant that severe hemophiliacs using clotting-factor concentrates were potentially exposed to tens of thousands of donors a year. Moreover, any given donor may potentially expose approximately one hundred persons. Hemophiliacs would be at highest risk, they said, but there was already a blood-transfused victim. In San Francisco, an infant had received a platelet transfusion from a man who subsequently was diagnosed as having AIDS. "Others can be anticipated." The donor was later tracked down. The baby died.

Dr. Olaf Krassnitzky, a former senior official with the Canadian Red Cross, says that after the January 1983 meeting in Atlanta there was no doubt that HIV was in the blood supply and would result in deaths of blood-transfused patients. But some officials demanded proof of danger to the public before they would act. "The argument that there was no scientific proof was the most awful red herring I've ever heard," Krassnitzky said in November 1993. "The argument must be: is there a risk to public health? And if there is sufficient association that the risk points to HIV, then action has to be taken."

Dr. Michelle Brill-Edwards of the Bureau of Human Prescription Drugs, a parallel office to the Bureau of Biologics in the federal Health Department, says proof is not necessary for action to be taken to protect public safety. The procedure followed in both bureaus would be the same in case of a health hazard, she says.

"If a pharmacist notified us that there's a bottle labelled digoxin but in fact contains penicillin, we'll go into a full alert on that for one darn bottle. There's a whole flurry: how did this happen? Go back and check the manufacturer's log books to look at what batch was going through. Could this be worse? Could there be thousands of bottles out there? And what's going to happen to people who should be on digoxin who are now taking penicillin? There's a procedure for that called the Health Hazard Procedure. Where are these people, when the highest authority on the globe [the World Health Organization] comes out in early 1983 and says: 'This fatal illness is blood-borne, by the way.' The whole response was totally muted."

Brill-Edwards says there are principles to be adhered to when managing risks and health hazards. "You weigh probabilities, but you don't ask for certainties. If it's four o'clock in the morning and I hear somebody trying to get in the front door, I don't wait until I see a guy with a gun standing in my bedroom. I call 911 as quick as I can. In public health, you don't wait for the body counts.

"It's absolute trash that you wait for scientific proof in dealing with health hazards. You don't. The whole point is that you prevent the tragedy from happening and the proof comes down the road. And if you never get the proof, if you don't have deaths, so much the better."

Most authorities seem to agree. Justice Horace Krever asked a Red

Cross official in September 1994 for a view on whether it was appropriate to wait for "proof beyond a reasonable doubt" before correcting a problem. A lot of bad things could happen while you were waiting for proof, the judge remarked. Michel Hebert, medical director of the Quebec Red Cross centre, agreed.

The U.S. Public Health Service recommended in March 1983 that persons with symptoms suggestive of AIDS and in high-risk groups should refrain from donating blood or plasma.

But early reports on the number of U.S. AIDS cases noted that less than 1 per cent were transfusion-related. That was the figure that caught the eye of optimists — and there were many — who chose to ignore the warnings. One study in the *New England Journal of Medicine* admitted the number of cases of transfusion-associated AIDS was small. But it also noted ominously that the transfused had received their blood between 1979 and early 1982, "when AIDS prevalence was much lower."

Around this time, many doctors were saying the chances of a hemophiliac contracting AIDS through blood were "one in a million." It's striking how many times that phrase crops up both in documents and in anecdotes told by the victims themselves. It may have been wishful thinking or just a handy cliché. But even in 1983, the proponents of that line would have needed a refresher course in math. In August 1983, Alan Brownstein told a U.S. congressional committee that 16 of 20,000 hemophiliacs had AIDS. It was, granted, a tiny minority — one out of 1,250. But risk increased with severity of hemophilia — for the severe cases it was one in 500.

Already, fear of AIDS was having tragic fallout on hemophiliacs and their families. Parents were wondering how close they and their non-hemophiliac kids should be to their hemophiliac children. Some did not want to send their kids to hemophiliac summer camps, fearing exposure to infected playmates. Spouses were afraid of having sex. There had been complaints from workplaces by people who were afraid to sit beside hemophiliac workmates. These complaints were being voiced in Canada as well as in the United States.

Physicians, blood-bank authorities, and government officials who downplayed the risk of HIV-AIDS transmission through blood often seized on the low infection rates among hemophiliacs to support their views. Some doctors hinted that infected hemophiliacs were in fact concealing their sexual leanings or drug abuse, and that those clandestine activities were the true cause of infection. Others argued that some unknown combination of factors, or multiple injections of concentrates, set off the inexorable march to AIDS. This did not explain the occurrences among mild hemophiliacs or surgery patients. A common view was that the presence of HIV antibodies in blood-product users did not necessarily mean AIDS was inevitable, just that there had been some exposure.

Even organizations representing hemophiliacs came late to the table. Despite Brownstein's forthright talk about the risk, the National Hemophilia Foundation continued to urge use of concentrates. An advisory late in 1983 from the National Hemophilia Foundation in the United States, for example, said that "only a fraction of 1 per cent of all hemophiliacs had contracted AIDS and no common lots have been identified among those who have the disease. This strongly suggests that the great majority of people with hemophilia are not susceptible to AIDS." The advice seemed at odds with the vigorous pitch Brownstein had made to Congress. Ironically, the advisory was issued after a recall of Cutter Laboratories Factor VIII and Factor IX, which occurred after a recently deceased blood donor was identified as having AIDS.

In Canada, not everyone was so dismissive. Chris Tsoukas, Hanna Strawczynski, and other Montreal doctors had begun their own study of "impaired cellular immunity" in October 1982 after hypothesizing hemophiliacs were vulnerable. The findings were reported a year later in the *Canadian Medical Association Journal*. Severe hemophiliacs may be at high risk for AIDS, they concluded. Four of thirty-four patients tested had "generalized lymphadenopathy."

"It is reasonable to postulate that another agent, as yet undefined, is transmitted in the Factor VIII preparations and is responsible for the observed immune abnormalities," they wrote. Hemophiliacs should be monitored for the development of opportunistic infections and malignant diseases. They, too, suggested that as concentrates were made from blood pooled from many donors, hemophiliacs would be at high risk.

The first Canadian hemophiliac death from AIDS occurred on March 31, 1983. He was Artibano Milito, a twenty-nine-year-old mill worker who died in New Westminster, British Columbia. The cause of death, according to information registered with the Federal Centre for AIDS, was toxoplasmosis, an infection of the brain that has killed many AIDS patients.

The emerging controversy over whether AIDS could be transmitted through blood was played out at an inquest into Milito's death. It was revealed that the month before he died, surgery for Milito had been cancelled because of the fear of transmitting AIDS to the patient. As a hemophiliac, Milito would have required large amounts of clotting concentrates. "The Red Cross is not releasing quantities unless it is an emergency because of the danger of transmitting AIDS," wrote Dr. Michael Noble, a blood specialist at New Westminster's Royal Columbian Hospital, on February 25, 1983. But for Milito, it was already too late.

At the inquest, held a year and a half after Milito died, an epidemiologist opined that the risk of contracting AIDS through blood transfusions or blood products was "almost zero for the average Canadian." Hemophiliacs were clearly not average Canadians.

In 1983, standard advice to hemophiliacs was to ignore the risk of HIV infection and to treat their bleeds. Severe bleeding was still the largest cause of death among this group, they were reminded. Those who raised concerns, including some in the media, were dismissed as alarmist.

This business-as-usual approach was affirmed in a May 1983 statement published in a hemophilia newsletter by Dr. Roslyn Herst of Toronto. She happened at the time to be wearing two hats—chair of Hemophilia Ontario's Medical and Scientific Advisory Committee and deputy medical director of the Toronto region Red Cross. Herst noted that while hemophiliacs had been identified as a risk group in the United States, "at the time of writing there had been no reports of hemophiliacs with AIDS in Canada. None of the approximately thirty cases of AIDS reported to date in Canada have been related to transfusion." She was mistaken — the death of Artibano Milito had already occurred.

"It should be stressed," Herst emphasized in capital letters, "that in hemophilia the risks of life-threatening or crippling bleeding episodes outweigh the potential risks associated with transfusion. Significant bleeding episodes must be adequately treated."

Then Herst appeared to challenge some of the alternatives suggested by the CHS national medical advisors, led by Dr. Strawczynski. "Consideration should be given to the most appropriate transfusion product for a particular individual. While the National MSAC recommendations suggest that the use of cryoprecipitate or exclusive use of products from Canadian plasma reduces the risk of exposure to AIDS, firm evidence for this is not available. Plasma source of product should not interfere with the decision to treat."

Herst also complained about media coverage of the spread of AIDS, calling it "alarmist and somewhat distorted." Hemophiliacs should not hesitate to infuse, she asserted.

The refrain about the alarmist media was not confined to Canada, or even to North America. The British newspaper *The Mail on Sunday* warned in May 1983 that tainted clotting factor was being imported from the United States and could transmit AIDS to British hemophiliacs. Treating physicians hauled the newspaper before the British Press Council. The council ruled later that summer that the paper had reported the threat in "extravagant and alarmist terms" and was "unacceptably sensational." Three years later, with 1,200 British blood-transfused patients infected, the newspaper was able to note, with grim satisfaction, that it had not been alarmist and its warnings had gone unheeded. "To warn and alarm is one of the first functions of a campaigning newspaper," the editors wrote.

It's significant that some hemophiliacs told Justice Horace Krever's inquiry in 1994 that they learned more about the peril from the media in the early 1980s than they did from their doctors or their own volunteer society.

In September 1983, Dr. Strawczynski issued an AIDS update for hemophiliacs. She noted that as of June there were fourteen American hemophiliacs with AIDS, two Canadians, and two Europeans. But, she said, the cause of AIDS was "still unknown" and there was no proof of transmission in blood. She did not mention the French discovery of LAV, but said the recommendations she had made in the previous February were still "fully endorsed."

Across Montreal, however, a doctor at Hôpital Ste-Justine was postulating that blood was the medium for transmission of the virus. In a letter in the *New England Journal of Medicine* on September 1, 1983, Dr. Normand Lapointe referred to a French-Canadian infant who had received two transfusions after birth, one from a donor later found to be HIV-positive. The baby exhibited similar symptoms to two children from the West Indies whose parents had abnormal systems. "These observations suggest common features with the syndrome described in adults and point to an agent or agents transmissible by blood and able to induce considerable immunosuppression, leading to death despite present-day medical therapy," Lapointe wrote.

Meanwhile, American hemophilia specialists unanimously approved a recommendation in October 1983 that concentrate be recalled if it contained material from an individual with AIDS or from anyone who "in the best medical judgment of the manufacturers, has characteristics strongly suggestive of AIDS." The U.S. foundation continued to urge hemophiliacs to maintain their prescribed use of concentrate or cryoprecipitate.

Hemophilia Society officials were watching developments south of the border with increasing alarm. Jo-Anne Harper, program director of the Ontario chapter, expressed her concern in a memo to national office in November 1983. "I believe that the chances of a recall happening in Canada as a result of a donor having AIDS are large, and it is only a matter of time until it happens."

The dilemma faced by hemophiliacs was expressed during an October 1983 meeting among Ontario Health Minister Keith Norton, representatives of the Ontario Hemophilia Society, and members of the AIDS Committee of Toronto. The hemophiliacs pointed out that AIDS was a life-threatening disease, but for members of their group "the fear of AIDS" was also life-threatening. Hemophiliacs were the only AIDS-affected group that could not modify their behaviour to reduce the risk of contracting AIDS, they noted. "All advice to hemophiliacs has been aimed to encourage them to continue their risk-inducing behaviour."

By December 1983, there were 2,952 AIDS cases in the United States, and 31 were being investigated as having occurred from blood transfusions. The spreading disease was starting to make converts out of previous non-believers. In an editorial in the *Annals of Internal Medicine* in January 1984, Dr. Joseph Bove of the Yale School of Medicine wrote, with a healthy dollop of understatement, that there was now "substantial evidence that transfusion-related AIDS does occur." A year earlier, Bove — also an official of the American Association of Blood Banks — had argued that evidence of the spread of AIDS through blood was lacking. Now, he said, doctors had to weigh the risks of transfusions against the expected benefits, and use them only if they are "unquestionably indicated."

By that time, there was enough known about AIDS to make some protective judgments in treatment. Blood products were clearly a possible medium for AIDS transmission, and hemophiliacs and transfused patients were at risk. Pooled products had a greater adverse impact on the immune system than single-donor ones. Even without isolation of the virus, logic would suggest that blood consumers should reduce their use of pooled concentrates.

Early in 1983, suggestions were made on how to block the HIV virus from entering the blood system in the first place. Some American blood bankers warned in January 1983 that blood from high-risk groups should not be used. They weren't completely convinced of the danger, however, and qualified their warning by saying evidence was "unproven, incomplete, and inconclusive." The same month, the National Hemophilia Foundation asked for measures to screen out high-risk groups, especially gay men, noting that one California firm, Alpha, bluntly asked potential donors if they had sex with other men. The commercial companies in the United States agreed, but the voluntary blood banks refused. The Canadian Red Cross then requested that members of high-risk groups — promiscuous gays, intravenous drug users, and Haitians — voluntary exclude themselves from donating. But the Red Cross, afraid that potential donors might believe they could contract HIV from giving their blood, kept the request low key. In March 1983, Dr. Roger Perrault, the Red Cross national director of blood services, said blood collected from high-risk donors was "not to be singled out at the moment."

Some gay community leaders were taking action to protect the blood supply without being asked. In Vancouver, especially, gays were active in urging caution, and this was true in some other cities as well. Regional Red Cross directors in some parts of the country were also anxious to improve donor screening.

But the national Red Cross seemed to crawl on the donor screening measure. According to Krassnitzky, Dr. John Derrick, the Red Cross advisor on regulatory affairs and manufacturing practices, was frustrated by the slow acceptance of donor screening in Canada.

"Once in a while he would walk into my office and complain," says Krassnitzky, one of several senior officials since fired by the Red Cross. "He'd say, 'Roger is not moving on this. We've got to push him.' He was totally frustrated with Perrault not moving." Derrick had gone to New York and brought back information on a voluntary donor-screening plan that was going on with the cooperation of the gay community.

Derrick may have backed better screening of blood donors, but he was much more reluctant to accept the concept that HIV transmitted through blood products was the cause of AIDS.

In July 1984, Derrick threw a bunch of numbers together in an article published in the *Canadian Medical Association Journal* and concluded that the frequency of transfusion-associated AIDS in the United States was one case per 500,000 transfusions. That was "a figure not greatly different from that for the general frequency of AIDS in the entire population." In Canada, Derrick added, no cases of AIDS as an outcome of transfusion therapy had been reported.

Hemophiliacs, he said, were eight hundred times more likely to be infected by AIDS than other transfusion patients, but he downplayed the rate of infection among them: "For every patient with hemophilia who has received these commercial concentrates and who has contracted AIDS, there are at least seven or eight hundred others receiving concentrates from the same lots who have not contracted the syndrome, in both the United States and Canada. Obviously, there must be significant factors other than the coagulation factor preparations that determine whether a patient receiving coagulation factor concentrates will contract AIDS."

Derrick also chided those doctors who proposed the use of cryoprecipitate in preference to concentrates, citing an article in the same issue about one of two Canadian hemophiliacs who had AIDS. In that case, a twenty-five-year-old hemophiliac treated in Toronto had developed AIDS after being treated "mainly" with cryoprecipitate. The man had switched to concentrates when he had adverse reactions to the older product. Derrick blamed the infection on cryoprecipitate.

"At this stage of AIDS research," wrote Derrick, "it should be emphasized that it is still not known whether the retrovirus is the causative agent of AIDS, whether other host co-factors are required in order for AIDS to develop, or even whether the presence of the retrovirus in a person signifies that he or she is capable of transmitting AIDS. It remains difficult to decide what additional action can presently be taken to further improve the safety of hemotherapy in Canada."

Derrick's article left the impression that there were no alternatives to defend blood users against the dire threat of AIDS. But alternatives did exist. In fact, research had already produced yet another alternative. Almost another year would pass, however, before Canadian hemophiliacs were able to receive it.

In 1993, Ken Poyser's grim message stood in stark contrast to the jubilation he had expressed twelve years earlier. "In 1983 our wings were clipped," he wrote in a fortieth-anniversary edition of *Hemophilia Today*. "Our joy was short-lived. Our freedom to live with less fear of illness or death was a short delight. A new threat entered into our community — a deadly killer, AIDS. I have lost many friends, colleagues I worked with, many who shared our joy, who dreamed our dreams, who desired a cure for hemophilia. Now we need a cure for both diseases."

DENISE ORIEUX

A member of the Canadian Hemophilia Society for more than thirty years, Denise Orieux may know better than anyone the price tainted blood has exacted on the blood-dependent community. The wiry, blonde woman is mother of three grown sons. The two younger brothers are HIV-positive hemophiliacs. Her work as the CHS Toronto and Central Ontario HIV-AIDS co-ordinator has brought her into contact with many more. A small quilt above her desk is decorated with fifty-two small angels, each representing someone she knew who has died of AIDS.

A self-described "tough old broad," she served as provincial president first in Manitoba and then in Ontario. For years, her watchword was trust.

"If anyone did anything for me or for any of the hemophiliacs, I was always so grateful. I trusted the doctors. I trusted the government. I even got politically involved with government to make sure I was out there making my contribution to society. I was not asleep. So people might say: 'You of all people should have known better.' But I didn't."

Orieux is a grassroots person. She says that once she gave her first talk on behalf of hemophiliacs, she just couldn't be shut up. Friends would hide behind the cornflakes displays in the supermarket because she'd be after them to donate blood.

In 1980, she dropped out of the Society for a while because she felt it had become cliquish. "It wasn't my down-to-earth, let's-go-hold-Mrs.-So-and-so's-hand society anymore. People peacocking around! But even then, I trusted. I might not have liked their silliness, but I trusted they would look after my needs as a member."

She kept in touch through the newsletters — the national society and the medical advisors saying everything was fine, that there was nothing wrong with the blood supply.

"I think this hurt me more than anything. You might say, 'What in the world are you doing back in the Society?' But you come back when something needs to be shaken up. I feel guilty because I didn't stick it out and question what they were doing. The doctors were saying everything was fine. I really did trust them. And it's not nice to break people's trust."

Her hemophiliac sons, Gregory and Martin, were raised not to use their condition as an excuse for missing school or feeling sorry for themselves. She says now she may have been an overly tough parent: "Had I known that they were both going to be infected with HIV, sometimes I think I wouldn't have pushed them so much. Mind you, they say to me, 'You were really good for us.' I adore them, and the thought that they might not be with me much longer is very hard.

"Sometimes I think my sons have given me a gift. There is a part of me that has developed through this that is so unconditional. I find that I am able to do things for people who are HIV-positive that I never thought I would be able to do. I can sit by a bed and wait for a last breath, and be aware of the special privilege of being there with someone when they take that last breath. I have never suffered so much. I have never experienced such deep sorrow, but it goes hand in hand with the understanding you get also."

Orieux says she is angry, but not interested in money because there can be no price on her children — they can never be replaced.

"With me, it's about the government of Canada, the prime minister, standing up in the House and saying: 'We apologize to all of these persons. We made a mistake and we're sorry.' I need that. I need for them to say they're sorry because they really screwed up!"

The blame for the saga of contaminated blood starts with the federal government's Bureau of Biologics, says Orieux. When the Bureau received word from the U.S. Centers for Disease Control in the summer of 1982 that there were infected American hemophiliacs, they should have acted.

"Our kids weren't infected in 1982. If anybody said to me, 'Well, we need proof,' I'd say, 'Would you take a chance? Would people who sell baby food take a chance?' They passed the buck. I can understand the Bureau of Biologics wanting some advice, but are they all morons with no balls? If somebody screams in the Maritimes that there's something wrong with tuna, it's off the shelves so fast because it's political. It could affect a lot of people. If the CDC was so concerned that they phoned the Bureau and told them, you pay attention to something like that. You don't start passing the buck. Who the hell makes the decisions up there? Nobody. That has to change. Now they are all grabbing for who's going to control what. And the band plays on!"

Orieux's sons Martin and Gregory are more like best buddies than brothers, she says. Martin, the younger one, now in his late twenties, was six-foot-two with bulging muscles when he found out he was HIV-positive. Wasting syndrome, diarrhea, and infections have taken a toll, and every muscle is atrophied. A music lover who won awards in high school for singing and drama, Martin wanted to go into audio-visual and sound effects as a career until he lost his hearing after a bout of meningitis in 1990.

Denise wants to have Martin fitted with a $15,000 hearing device so he can listen to music before he dies. But one delay follows another. She believes excuses are being made by medical authorities who have decided it would be a waste to use the aid on a patient who is HIV-positive.

"If it's the $15,000, heck, why not tell him? He could have gone to the States and bought one. He doesn't mind. He's got the money. We would hawk our homes, for crying out loud, and sell everything, just to make sure he could hear something. I've been praying for four years that something would happen so he could hear before he died."

Martin's brother Gregory is thirty and is described as a Mr. Health type. He's very careful what he eats and follows many of the health-conscious guidelines established for the gay community.

A few years ago, Orieux got a call from Gregory after midnight. He had rushed Martin, who was totally disoriented, into hospital where the younger man had suffered convulsions. When Denise got there, Gregory was sitting in a chair, sobbing.

"Oh, Mom, he hasn't even had a chance for a relationship. He's only getting over being shy and noticing girls. And he's never going to be able to have a life like that. He's going to die."

Denise thought, "My God, here is this kid who is in the same boat, with HIV, and he's taken all that responsibility for his brother."

Denise Orieux likes to say she has lost her naivety, but has regained her innocence.

"This disease has so overwhelming an effect because my sons are going to die. And at the same time, it's like something has been lifted. It's like all of a sudden I have brains in my head. It's like all of a sudden I've regained my innocence. It's like all of a sudden there is beauty in the flowers. And the rain is falling on the dirt and you can smell the earth. Every moment is precious. I have no time to waste on bullshit.

"I'm not sorry I had my sons. I was never once sorry I had sons with hemophilia. For their sakes, I wish they hadn't had it. But no, they haven't made my life miserable. They have given and given and given. It's like my hemophiliac friends. I can make a retreat with your wife, and she can hold me in her arms and we, as two mothers, can share some-thing that is so deep, so profound, so genuine. You get forty-eight women together and you don't hear one nasty word. The room is filled with compassion and love. This is my family. This is where my support is. If I'm going to die and have a reward, it will be because the people within the hemophiliac family have been my salvation. They have taught me all about love, about tolerance, about patience."

Chapter 4

CONFUSION AND DENIAL

*"Common sense said the downside is so great and the
upside is so positive that if it happened to work, why are
we hesitating for the few cents extra?"*

KEN POYSER, FORMER PRESIDENT OF THE CANADIAN HEMOPHILIA SOCIETY

Once the nightmarish virus that caused AIDS had been identified, scientists turned their attention in 1984 to ways to eradicate it from the blood supply. Heat treatment had been shown to be partially successful against hepatitis viruses, so why not try it against this new plague? There were doubters, however, who argued that the evidence in favour of heat treatment was inconclusive and that the treatment might destroy vast quantities of blood products, pushing up costs. The resistance put Canada in the back seat when efforts were made to acquire the new products.

Acceptable evidence for most authorities came in September 1984, when the British medical journal *Lancet* reported an experiment conducted in the California laboratories of the blood-fractionating company Cutter. Mouse retroviruses had been added to human plasma and this was processed into the coagulant Factor VIII. The retrovirus survived the manufacturing procedure. But then the Factor VIII had been subjected to heat for several hours. It was discovered after heat treatment of 68 degrees Celsius for ninety-six hours that no retrovirus was detectable. The researchers concluded that prolonged heating at this temperature should be used to manufacture the clotting factor.

The experiment was repeated by the Centers for Disease Control in Atlanta, and the conclusion reached that HIV would be killed by the application of heat. The findings were reported October 26, 1984, in the *Morbidity and Mortality Weekly Report*. The National Hemophilia Foundation in the United States, keeping a watchful eye on the CDC work, called for use of heat-treated product in mid-October.

News of the heat-treatment process quickly spread. Even before the *Lancet* article was published and before the Americans opted for the change, the Canadian Hemophilia Society had started efforts to obtain heat-treated products. At a meeting on September 10, 1984, with representatives of the four major suppliers to the Canadian market (Cutter, Connaught, Armour, and Baxter-Hyland), CHS officials said they were very worried that heat-treated products were available in the United States, but had apparently not been procured for Canada. The CHS decided to express its grave concern at an October meeting of the advisory sub-committee to the Canadian Blood Committee.

Although some resisters said what worked in the test tube might not necessarily work in the body, the studies prompted a rapid changeover in the United States to heat-treated products. Canadian hemophiliacs were sideswiped by this transition. One effect was that an existing shortage of concentrates was apparently made even worse. American producers began destroying non-heat-treated lots and directed new heat-treated products to their domestic consumers. Some other countries recalled untreated factor and put an embargo on untreated U.S. concentrates.

At a meeting on October 11, 1984, with Bill Mindell, chair of the Ontario Hemophilia Society's Factor Products Committee, Dr. Derek Naylor of the Canadian Red Cross cited several reasons for a growing shortage of blood products. Normally, there was a two-month supply across Canada. This inventory had fallen to two weeks. The supply plan for the year was six to eight weeks behind schedule because of delivery delays due to testing by the federal Bureau of Biologics. Two lots of Cutter product had been destroyed because some donors might have been infected with hepatitis. Mindell reports that the Bureau had put in extra testing or quarantine to be sure. And Connaught

Laboratories, the sole Canadian producer, was struggling with major long-term production difficulties.

Furthermore, Naylor said, introduction of heat-treated products in the United States had reduced the amount of regular concentrate in the inventories of U.S. fractionators. And increased surveillance and destruction of lots found to be contaminated by AIDS had reduced supplies.

Naylor did not mention a possible shift to heat-treated factors or their potential availability in Canada. He and other influential voices in the Red Cross still had reservations about the now-duplicated findings in the United States on heat-treated products. Mindell says today the new heat-processed concentrates cost 40 to 45 per cent more, and that Naylor and his colleague John Derrick felt it was a "big money grab" by the manufacturers for a product that was not particularly effective. (That view was repeated at the Krever hearings in Edmonton in April 1994 by Dr. Jean-Michel Turc, who referred to a "marketing ploy.")

When the first North American heat-treated products were introduced in 1983, Derrick had expressed reservations about how effective they were against hepatitis. Those reservations carried over to the new claims. But Mindell says senior Red Cross officials were also concerned that the heating process might lead to the development of inhibitors in patients. Inhibitors are antibodies to the transfused factor that develop in about 10 per cent of severe hemophiliacs, blocking the effectiveness of the injected material. The inhibitors, capable of destroying not only transfused material but what little factor the patient's own body produces, are a serious development because they put hemophilia treatment for the unfortunate patient back to the Dark Ages of the 1950s.

"It was certainly a theoretical concern," Mindell said in May 1994. Heat-treated products, he says, were a new toy. "That was a very strongly held view in the Red Cross, and I didn't find anyone else pushing it. It was a watch-and-wait thing for everybody in the business.

"They just never really let go of that, even when the evidence started coming in about the HIV destruction. They were more worried about the inhibitors than about the impact of HIV on the concentrates. And naive or foolish as that may sound, it was a sincerely held view."

If inhibitors were a concern, this was not reflected in the documents. When Naylor and Derrick co-authored an article resisting introduction of heat-treated products for Hemophilia Ontario's newsletter in October 1984, they didn't mention inhibitors once.

But some members of the Hemophilia Society harboured doubts as well. While accepting that heat-treated products were safer, Mindell himself remained to be convinced they were the solution to the AIDS puzzle. And even when the National Hemophilia Foundation in the United States strongly urged treaters to switch to heat-treated concentrates in mid-October 1984, it added the qualification that "protection against AIDS is yet to be proven."

In hindsight, one wonders why it was so difficult to move the doubters and why it took so long for heat-treated blood derivatives to gain wide acceptance. Heat treatment had been used in Europe for some time to halt the spread of hepatitis B virus through blood, although no company guaranteed it would be totally effective. Early in 1984, according to Canadian Hemophilia Society documents, no fewer than seven companies were producing heat-treated products. California-based Baxter-Hyland had received a licence from the Canadian government for its heat-treated product in November 1983. If these processed products could kill one virus, why not another?

One European study matching results of heated versus non-heated products in so-called virgin (previously untreated) hemophiliacs had begun in December 1982 and concluded in June 1984. French, Italian, and Belgian researchers — including Luc Montagnier, the discoverer of LAV — began an experiment in which a group of eighteen hemophiliacs were given heat-purified blood products made by Baxter-Hyland. A control group of twenty-nine, also previously untreated patients (or PUPS, as some medical authorities referred to them), was provided with non-heated products. When the experiment ended in the summer of 1984, none of those given the heat-treated products showed signs of HIV antibodies. But five of the unfortunate twenty-nine in the control group were seropositive. The results were not published until February 1985, and by then most experts believed that heat treatment would destroy the virus. In retrospect, it might appear that those in the control group were treated like guinea pigs, but when the test began no one could have said with conviction whether or not the groups were at equal risk.

Others had previously suggested heat purification of clotting concentrates might prove to be effective. The question was asked by Gilbert White and Henry Lesesne in the *Annals of Internal Medicine* in March 1983. "Heated preparations of Factor VIII that are reported to have greatly reduced hepatitis B risk have been described. Will the same treatment inactivate the acquired immunodeficiency syndrome virus?" they asked.

In Canada, a feeler about heat-treated products had come a year before *Lancet* published results of the Cutter trial. In mid-1983, Dr. Hanna Strawczynski, then chairperson of the medical advisory committee of the Canadian Hemophilia Society, wrote to the Red Cross about heat-treated products. Strawczynski, concerned about the use of commercial American products, had wondered why some parts of Canada, including the two largest cities, were using so much commercially purchased blood from the United States as opposed to volunteer-sourced. There had long been concerns that products made from purchased American blood were more likely to be contaminated. Strawczynski had attended the National Hemophilia Foundation meeting on January 14, 1983, at which officials of the Centers for Disease Control warned of contamination in the blood supply and American hemophilia specialists suggested alternatives to Factor VIII use. John Derrick, the Red Cross advisor on regulatory affairs and good manufacturing practices, had also attended that meeting. While Strawczynski emerged from the session with concerns about unlimited use of concentrates, Derrick apparently leaned towards the opinion of American blood bankers who were skeptical of warnings that AIDS was being spread by bad blood.

Derek Naylor told Strawczynski that patients in the Montreal area needed supplements of U.S. commercial product because hematologists were aggressively treating hemophiliacs with prophylactic doses, designed to stop bleeds before they start. In Toronto, the failure of Canadian-owned Connaught Laboratories to produce efficiently from plasma collected from Ontario volunteers had compelled the importation of less-safe American products.

Naylor's letter also referred to heat-treated products: "Endorsement of the use of this product would further compromise the goals of national self-sufficiency in view of the reduction in yields caused by the heat-treatment process."

Naylor and Derrick summarized their doubts about heat treatment in an article published in the October 26, 1984, newsletter of Hemophilia Ontario, the provincial branch of the volunteer society.

The national Blood Transfusion Service of the Red Cross had decided against production or distribution of heat-treated products then being made by four American suppliers. Naylor and Derrick wrote that there was "inconclusive evidence that such products . . . are free of virus infectivity." Moreover, Canadian fractionators — then Connaught and Winnipeg's Rh Institute — were unlicensed to produce heat-treated products. The Red Cross doctors also argued that yields of Factor VIII can be up to 25 per cent lower than with the non-treated product, which could mean worsening shortages of the coagulants. Economic considerations were also cited — the new products would be more costly. (One American authority put the cost at 16 cents a unit compared with 12 cents. For a fairly typical infusion of 800 units, the cost would be US$32 per dose higher.)

The article reported that almost half of Canada's Factor VIII concentrate still had to be imported because yields were already low by current fractionation methods. This was another important reason for the cautious approach when the evidence for heat treatment was "inconclusive." Further, for every North American hemophiliac who had come down with AIDS (to that time) there were several hundred using the same products who had not. "This almost certainly means that other predisposing host factors are probably involved."

Long-term controlled clinical trials were needed to determine the efficacy of heat treatment in reducing viral transmission, the authors argued. So, "no recommendation can be made that presently licensed heat-treated products should be used." Had that attitude prevailed, hundreds more blood users might have been infected.

A last-minute editor's note, however, stood out in stark contrast. "We have just learned that the use of heat-treated Factor VIII has been recommended by the National Hemophilia Foundation." In fact, the American group's medical advisory committee had made the recommendation on October 13, two days after Mindell and Naylor met.

In that light, the timing of the published article seems peculiar. Within days, Derrick's name was on a memo to the advisory subcommittee of the Canadian Blood Committee. As evidence grows that retroviruses are vulnerable to relatively mild heat treatment, "there may well be greater justification for use of heat-treated Factor VIII concentrate," Derrick wrote on October 30. His public message to hemophiliacs was sharply at odds with the view expressed privately to colleagues.

Even before Naylor and Derrick sent in their article, there had been two other requests for heat-processed products on behalf of Canadian hemophiliacs. On October 15, Dr. Man-Chiu Poon had written Naylor urging him, in light of the emerging evidence and action taken in the United States, that the Red Cross reconsider its stance towards heat-treated products. Poon, co-author in March 1983 of one of the first American reports on AIDS in hemophiliacs when he was in Alabama, was now practicing in Calgary and a member of the Hemophilia Society's medical and scientific advisory committee, or MSAC. Poon had learned through American connections that seropositivity among American hemophiliacs was believed to be about 70 per cent. That was an alarming figure, especially since half of the factor concentrates Canadians used were American-sourced.

Poon noted blood products had been heat treated with "minimal decrease" of Factor VIII potency. He urged Naylor to look at these developments "very carefully and objectively," and warned that Canadian hemophiliacs would press for the new products when the word spread.

Then Bill Rudd, a former CHS national president and chairman of its Blood Resources Committee, announced at an October 19 meeting between the Red Cross and the CHS that shortages of concentrates were critical. He deplored the lack of communication between the Red Cross and the patients who were reliant on the products. Rudd, who had already pointed out in a September meeting that some American centres were using heat-treated material for small children, called for more products to be obtained from the most competent and effective fractionators. He didn't care whether they were Canadian or American and also asked that heat-treated products be obtained in preference to non-treated.

The Red Cross answer was to repeat that Canadian fractionators were not licensed to produce heat-treated products, and to suggest "national self-sufficiency would be compromised" if there was a preference for the new heat-purified coagulants. But given the choice between imports of heat-treated products or domestically produced untreated clotting factor, there's no doubt Canadian hemophiliacs would have opted for the margin of safety. Red Cross officials apparently expected that choice, because they also argued that if users believed the more costly heat-treated products were safer — even though the evidence was inconclusive — they would all demand them.

There may not have been a Canadian manufacturer of heat-treated concentrates, but Baxter-Hyland had been given a licence by the Canadian government to sell a heat-processed product in November 1983, a year earlier. Baxter, however, does not seem to have been high on the Red Cross popularity list. The company had offered its product almost immediately after licensing in November as a protection against hepatitis B. "Unfortunately," the Red Cross now says, "the hepatitis B virus often survived the process, and the amount of Factor VIII produced was reduced substantially. In addition, the Baxter process produced Factor VIII that was much more expensive than other Factor VIII available at the time."

Stephen Vick, assistant national director for manufacturing, says today that the Red Cross reviewed Baxter's product in 1983 and rejected it on the grounds that it did not inactivate hepatitis B. "I think at the time it was viewed as more of a marketing gimmick than anything else. In hindsight, who knows?" he laughs. "But at the time it was not effective against hepatitis and that's why it wasn't selected. Who knows how things would have been otherwise?"

Vick notes that Baxter was the only North American company at the time offering heat-treated products. "They were touting it as 'somewhat effective' against hepatitis B. In their actual sales pitch, the 'somewhat' might have been dropped once or twice, but if you look at their written literature, which had to be accurate, it was 'somewhat effective'."

Baxter's first offer had come before heat treatment was shown to inactivate HIV. The company would make two other proposals later on.

Ken Poyser, another former CHS national president and the CHS representative to the advisory sub-group of the Canadian Blood Committee, reminded fellow committee members on October 30 that heat-treated concentrates had been available, as anti-hepatitis products, in the United States for two years. They had also been available in Europe since 1980. And they could have been made available in Canada, too.

Poyser had been pushing for the introduction of heat-treated products for two years. "I knew there was scientific evidence that showed heat treatment worked against hepatitis," he said in the spring of 1994. "If it worked against hepatitis, that made it a better product immediately in my mind. Why shouldn't we, as Canadian hemophiliacs, have the best treatment available?

"Secondly, I was given enough information to indicate that heat treatment worked against a lot of viruses. If it turned out it was a virus, there was a chance because heat treatment works against so many things. We had to reach for any chance possible at that time. Common sense said the downside is so great and the upside is so positive that if it happened to work, why are we hesitating over the few cents extra?"

Wark Boucher, then chief of the blood products division of the federal Bureau of Biologics, responded to Poyser, saying he did not recommend changeover to heat-treated factors. He, like Red Cross officials, wanted more proof that heat-treated products would solve the problem of blood contamination, and argued it would result in lost yields. The Bureau would not recommend a switch.

What Boucher was telling colleagues in the Bureau was quite different. In a memo dated October 4, 1984, about Cutter's heat-treated Factor VIII concentrate, Boucher wrote that the available information suggested heating might not destroy hepatitis B but "may be effective for inactivation of the human T-cell leukemia virus postulated to be the cause of AIDS." He concluded his memo to Dr. D. C. Pope, assistant director of the Bureau, with the following recommendation: "I see no objection to approval of the above Supplemental/New Drug Submission for the heat treatment of Factor VIII."

Now, senior representatives of both the Canadian Red Cross and the federal Health Department had privately accepted that heat treatment might work against the virus. In public, they were still demanding more proof.

The Red Cross's Roger Perrault, national director of the blood transfusion service, said Canadian-source plasma in the pipeline was ready to produce eight million units of clotting factor. He fretted that if a changeover was made to heat treatment, there would be a problem sorting out who should get the treated products. The construction of that dilemma wasn't good enough for some advisors to the Canadian Blood Committee. Dr. Martin Inwood, long an active supporter of the Canadian Hemophilia Society, and a representative of the Canadian Cancer Society both expressed concern over the conservative approach. There was still no discussion of urgent measures, even though this was the fourth time in a month that concerns had been raised by the CHS or people associated with it.

In late October the Canadian Red Cross dispatched a representative to a special session of the American Association of Blood Banks, at which use of heat-treated derivatives was endorsed. After the delegate returned, Derrick sent a memo on October 29 to Perrault. Cutter now had available a heat-treated product that inactivated retroviruses without affecting the potency of the product, he advised. For the Red Cross this was a turning point, but consumers of the blood products were still not home free. It would be at least six months before heat-treated concentrates would be distributed to Canadians.

Derrick now assumed that all but previously untreated hemophiliacs had already been exposed to the AIDS agent. His memo appears to discount any urgency in distribution, the Canadian Hemophilia Society argues, because Derrick may have believed it was too late for most hemophiliacs. The evidence was certainly strong by the fall of 1984 that large numbers already had compromised immune systems. Indeed, Health Canada had test results that indicated a majority of hemophiliacs might already be HIV-positive. Curiously, these shocking results became mired in the Health Department bureaucracy. On both sides of the border, it appeared, the vast majority of severe hemophiliacs — the most frequent users of concentrates — had been infected.

Pressure would be strong for use of the heat-processed products, Derrick predicted. He was still reluctant to accept the notion that heat treatment would reduce the spread of AIDS. His preference was to supplement Canadian-made non-treated products with U.S. heat-treated materials. Derrick also raised the question of how the new product would be shared out and urged a consensus conference where guidelines for distribution could be discussed. He made no suggestion that perhaps hemophiliacs should be tested for HIV to determine who was still negative and therefore could benefit from use of the heat-treated product. This omission may have resulted in the needless infection of many hemophiliacs.

Overnight, Red Cross authorities changed their minds and the federal regulator, the Bureau of Biologics, followed suit. The reversal happened suddenly, like the collapse of a house of cards. On October 31, Derrick acknowledged in a memo the efficacy of heat treatment. Cutter Laboratories received its Canadian licence for its heat-treated product on November 13, 1984. On November 16, the Bureau of Biologics announced its new stance in a telex to the eight suppliers or would-be suppliers of blood-clotting concentrates to Canada. It directed the replacement of non-treated products with virus-inactivating heat-treated products as soon as feasible. "We have informed the Canadian Red Cross that further reliance on AHF (anti-hemophilic factor) products that have not been heat-treated cannot be justified," the telex said pointedly.

Abruptly, the assumptions about blood products had changed and the shift led to a flurry of position papers, briefing notes, telexes, and meetings, all leading up to the consensus conference on December 10. Six days after the Bureau of Biologics' declaration that non-heat-treated concentrates could not be relied upon any longer, the executive of the Canadian Blood Committee met to consider the Hemophilia Society's request. There were no representatives of the consumer group present. Peter Glynn, assistant deputy minister of the Health Promotions Branch, asked if Cutter was in a position to supply Canada with heat-treated product. "The answer is yes, probably at any time (to be negotiated)," minutes of the November 22 meeting state.

Through a conference call, Roger Perrault suggested to the executive that introduction of the products be phased in "to avoid anxiety with hemophiliacs." Perrault also noted the impact on Canada's struggling fractionation industry would be significant — the goal of national self-sufficiency in blood products might be jeopardized.

Earlier that month, John Derrick had raised other concerns. It would cost about $300,000 more to buy heat-treated products in place of the old concentrates, he noted in a background paper. Derrick suggested that American fractionators, who were switching production entirely to heat-treated concentrates, might require a waiver releasing them from any damages arising from any of the old product they were providing to Canada.

There was continuing preoccupation with the future of the domestic blood-products industry. A November 28 briefing note prepared by the Canadian Blood Committee Secretariat for Health Minister Jake Epp referred to the longstanding problems of Connaught Laboratories, and said heat treatment could further delay Factor VIII preparation at Winnipeg's Rh Institute, which had been on target for a July 1985 start. As it happened, the Rh Institute had been experimenting with heat treatment of freeze-dried concentrates as early as the spring of 1984. The construction of a third Canadian producer, the Armand Frappier Centre in Montreal, had been delayed, too. "We have to keep in mind that Ministers of Health have approved the three above plants to ensure national self-sufficiency in blood products," it said.

There were three alternatives for Canadian manufacturers: to buy heat-treating technology from the United States, which would mean a four- to six-month wait before the products were available; to develop the technology, which would mean a six-month to one-year delay; or to withdraw from fractionation.

Another choice was contrary to the goal of national self-sufficiency: to buy the safer products from American fractionators. That option, which was selected, was not popular with the Canadian fractionators. At a meeting of the Blood Committee executive in January 1985, Bill Cochrane, the chairman of Connaught, called the decision of the Bureau of Biologics "good in essence but premature." "Even the hemophiliacs were not expecting such a decision at so early a date," he wrongly opined.

And what of hemophiliacs dependent on the products? "If the supply of heat-treated Factor VIII is not assured within a reasonable time, the hemophiliac community may feel inadequately protected," the briefing material suggested. A draft produced by the Secretariat had a warning: "Should events occur indicating that all efforts to protect hemophiliacs from infection by the causative agent had not been carried out, legal consequences could be very serious."

And the threat could spread beyond the hemophiliac community. "The isolation of HTLV-III from an apparently healthy person who subsequently developed AIDS has also added to concerns that a carrier state may exist in asymptomatic individuals who are healthy enough to be accepted as blood donors," said a Bureau of Biologics position paper prepared for the December 10 meeting.

The new products would take time to arrive. Meanwhile, deliveries of non-heat-treated products would continue from Cutter, Armour, and Connaught for months after the Bureau ordered heat treatment. Stephen Vick says those arrivals were part of the contracted supplies for the fiscal year, which ended in March 1985. The last non-heated commercial Armour product arrived in December 1984, Cutter's final non-heated commercial delivery was in February 1985, and Connaught supplied some as late as mid-April. Non-heated Factor VIII made by Cutter and Connaught from Canadian-collected Red Cross plasma also arrived as late as April.

"We were continuing to issue it until we had the heat-treated to replace it," says Vick. "But when the heat-treated came in we started to replace the non-heat-treated, and eventually had sufficient to replace it totally." Vick says no spot purchases of non-treated concentrates were made after the Bureau's directive. There was no spot purchasing of heat-treated products either, he adds, because the contracted supplies arranged early in 1985 were all the Red Cross could get.

But even when the long-awaited replacement products did arrive, documents show the distribution was slow. Old non-heated concentrates were sent out routinely to hemophiliacs while the safer ones sat on Red Cross shelves, purportedly for use in emergency. There was no apparent recognition that this, in fact, was the emergency.

The Bureau of Biologics had predicted the new products would be available within two to three months, in other words between mid-January and mid-February. But no supplies were obtained by the Red Cross before the planned December 10 conference at which distribution of the heat-processed product was to be discussed. The delay ensured that the Bureau's time estimate could not be achieved.

Within days of the Bureau's directive, the Red Cross, toughening its abrupt about-face, diverted all remaining fresh-frozen plasma produced in Canada in 1984 to Cutter. Connaught, however, was asked to continue producing non-treated factor from the plasma already delivered, until the end of March 1985.

The consensus conference of December 10, 1984, was attended by representatives from all interested parties. Rudd, an accounting firm partner from New Westminster, British Columbia, and Poyser represented the Canadian Hemophilia Society and had observer status. Both had argued forcefully for speedy replacement of non-heat-treated products by heat-processed. Dr. Robert Card, chairman of the CHS medical advisors, was also present.

Poyser forced himself into the discussion and argued vigorously for fast introduction of heat-treated products, but many of the score of participants felt the threat was exaggerated.

To Bob O'Neill, then the Society's Ontario chapter director, the conference was "pivotal." O'Neill says other "experts" dismissed the urgency of the situation and tried to convince Rudd that those pushing for the new concentrates were over-reacting. They also suggested there would be clotting-factor shortages if all the non-treated product was recalled. Many experts could not seem to accept that having the HIV antibody was fatal.

Others had no doubt that heat-treated products should be speedily introduced. Among them was Albert Friesen, executive director of Winnipeg's Rh Institute, who urged quick licensing of his university-based production facility. "Since this heat treatment does not present a hazard to the user and provides a supply of material which will almost certainly reduce the risk of exposure of hemophiliacs to live retroviruses, the use of heat-treated Factor VIII should begin as soon as possible," an institute backgrounder stated.

The key recommendation from the meeting, according to a joint statement from the Red Cross and the Canadian Hemophilia Society, was that introduction of heat-processed factor "could be accomplished before May 1985 with a period of transition from the use of non-heat-treated to the use of heat-treated products not exceeding eight weeks thereafter." In other words, the completion date for the changeover was to be July 1. During that eight weeks, both products would be used. The criteria by which patients would receive the heated and non-heated products would be decided by the Medical and Scientific Advisory Committee, the professionals who advised the lay members of the CHS.

In fact, there were nine recommendations on which consensus was reached that were incorporated in a final draft from the meeting. These were approved the next day by the executive of the Canadian Blood Committee. Among them was a request to the Bureau of Biologics to expedite licensing of heat-treatment concentrates and procedures; a recommendation that all Factor VIII in the plasma or cryoprecipitate stage be heat-treated; and that all Red Cross plasma be directed to fractionators licensed to heat-treat until Canadian manufacturers adopted the process. These fractionators, of course, were all located outside Canada.

But two other recommendations listed second and third in a first draft from the consensus meeting were oddly omitted from the final version. "Recommends that *only* [my emphasis] heat-treated Factor VIII be produced or purchased for use in Canada," said one. "That this conference agrees to the eventual exclusive use of heat-treated Factor VIII in Canada to be implemented as early as possible," said the second. The blood bureaucrats may have felt these explicit recommendations would tie their hands too much.

"Everybody who was involved in the meeting agreed to the plan," says O'Neill. "Nobody disagreed with the July 1, 1985, implementation, and both the Medical and Scientific Advisory Committee and the

Canadian Hemophilia Society went along with it. The question is, Were these people fully informed of the risk? [Federal officials] say nobody knew the extent of the risk. They did not know at that time that everybody who got the virus would get sick and die. And that's what they were telling Bill Rudd. I guess they didn't want to assume the worst."

That attitude was common at the time, says O'Neill, who now works at St. Paul's Hospital in Vancouver, the primary AIDS centre in that city. "I had a lot of conversations with John Derrick. He kept telling us we were over-reacting. We really didn't know. We were just trying to make the system safer. It's all a question of relative risk, whether they believed people who had a blood transfusion were at risk. They definitely believed the risk was low.

"In the summer of 1984, both the Red Cross and the government stated most hemophiliacs had been exposed to HIV, but they didn't believe that meant they would get AIDS. Hematologists were saying that if a person had antibodies they didn't know what that meant. There was a reluctance to admit not so much the transmission of HIV, but the transmission of AIDS. The Red Cross wanted to protect the image of the blood supply. They erred in that regard, but I don't know if they consciously decided [to ignore the risk]," says O'Neill.

Four days before the conference, a letter from Dr. Chris Tsoukas of Montreal had appeared in the *New England Journal of Medicine* saying that 56 per cent of concentrate-using Factor VIII hemophiliacs in a study had HIV antibodies. This backed up earlier evidence from both Canada and the United States that about half of hemophiliacs were already infected. This also meant that the other half were not, but no measures seem to have been advocated at the conference to protect them. Non-infected, severe hemophiliacs as a group appear to have been abandoned when decisions were made as to which patients were to receive the first limited supplies of the new heat-treated products.

A vital question is whether supplies available were enough to provide for non-infected severe hemophiliacs. If there were adequate quantities, as Dr. Rey Pagtakhan, a Winnipeg MP and physician, noted in the Commons sub-committee hearings of February 1993, severe hemophiliacs should also have been given the new products, "because to make a universal assumption that all of them must have been infected is a very summary conviction."

At the end of December 1984, an editorial appeared in the *Lancet* that gave a new urgency to the transition to heat-treated products. AIDS had turned up in apparently healthy HIV-positive mothers. If there had been any doubt before, the development showed these antibodies were unlike those in most other diseases and were "not necessarily protective." The *Lancet* predicted that a main immediate spinoff would be the large-scale development of antibody tests to exclude antibody-positive blood donors.

The *Lancet* sought to push any laggards who might still oppose the use of heat-purified concentrates. "It would be indefensible to allow prescription and home use of material known to be at risk from HTLV-III when apparently safer preparations are available."

Other recipients of blood products could be at risk, the editorial warned. "The safety considerations extend beyond hemophilia. All blood products must be reassessed in the light of these events. Plasminogen, fibrinogen, and other pooled blood and human tissue products must be regarded as potential hazards until proven otherwise."

Yet Bob O'Neill says Red Cross officials and many hematologists treating hemophiliacs wanted to believe that the risk of developing AIDS from HIV was not strong. In a memo written in 1988, O'Neill says that Derrick maintained as late as April 1985 that "in his mind it had not been proven that HIV has ever been transmitted through a blood donation."

"I call it institutional and professional denial," O'Neill said recently. "You like to believe you are helping them and you don't want to admit something is wrong. Don't ask me the psychological process behind it!"

Chapter 5

DELAYED RESPONSE

*"They were afraid that if they faced up to it, people would say,
'Gee, maybe there's something wrong with that stuff!' And sure
enough, there was something wrong with that stuff."*

TOM DREES, FORMER PRESIDENT OF ALPHA THERAPEUTICS, FEBRUARY 1994

Suspicion and controversy surround the chain of events after the December 1984 consensus conference. Once the federal government directed that heat-treated concentrates should be acquired as soon as feasible and the provinces agreed to pay, reliable and sufficient supplies had to be arranged for the country's hemophiliacs. The Red Cross was to negotiate contracts with suppliers outside Canada. A timetable was set out for distribution of the new products, and medical advisors to the Canadian Hemophilia Society were to draw up a list of priority recipients.

The Red Cross maintains it was simply unable to obtain supplies of the suddenly popular heat-treated products as 1984 drew to a close, but this is debatable. At least two American authorities who kept close watch on supplies at that period say that sufficient heat-treated factor would have been available for Canadians. There were also six European suppliers who might have had product and apparently went untapped. It may have been a matter of how much Canadian authorities were prepared to pay. David Page, past president of the Canadian Hemophilia Society, says what the Red Cross has failed to show is evidence of the effort it made to obtain heat-treated product.

But there's another angle to this dismal tale. The question arises: did the Red Cross deliberately drag its feet and time the introduction of the heat-treated products so that it could use up its complete inventory of the old, now-suspect concentrates?

A Red Cross list of its non-heated products as of December 1, 1984, shows that supplies on hand and deliveries expected of non-heated products would have lasted until May 1, 1985. So even before the experts had met to discuss the implementation date for the introduction of heat-treated products, Red Cross officials had likely made up their minds. Based on average weekly usage, May 1 would allow the Red Cross to dump virtually its complete stock of non-heated products before it would have to start doling out the safer — and more expensive — products.

This seems to have been a calculated decision. There is no expression of urgency to get the heat-treated materials out to consumers before May 1. Indeed, the concern expressed on the inventory list is a warning that if the inefficient Canadian producer Connaught failed to deliver its non-heated concentrates on time, the inventory might be depleted before May 1.

Page suggests the slow distribution pattern was not accidental. The inventory computes the weekly consumption rate of non-heat-treated products. "In reality, between May 1 and July 1 they had used up 95 per cent of the products they had in stock, all but a two-week supply," says Page. "The facts bear out that they were very successful in using up all the products. This document shows that there was some premeditation as to the amount of time it would take to use up these products."

Dr. Roger Perrault, then national director of the Blood Transfusion Service, told the executive of the Canadian Blood Committee on December 11, 1984, that as far as he was concerned, "the inventory has to be dealt with." Nobody at the consensus conference — and specifically the Hemophilia Society — had requested him to write off the inventory of non-heat-treated concentrates that were now deemed potentially unsafe.

The Health Department, too, apparently gave the go-ahead to the Red Cross to exhaust its stock of non-heated concentrates. Briefing notes for Dr. D. C. Pope of the Health Protection Branch dated November 27, 1987, say: "Earlier lots of these products already on the market were allowed to be used up." The Bureau of Biologics would have given the green light.

The Bureau had, indeed, been asked to allow distribution of non-heated products until sufficient heat-treated concentrates were available, according to Janice Hopkins, the executive director of the Health Protection Branch in early 1993. She says that request came from the Hemophilia Society's medical advisors. But it was made in November 1984, when the Bureau anticipated introduction of the new products by mid-January to mid-February. In fact, the first heat-processed concentrates were first distributed in May and the wholesale switch not made until July 1.

The Red Cross seemed determined to stick to its schedule regardless of the public peril. Producers had been barred from selling those non-heated coagulants in the United States and West Germany, but Canada's atmosphere in early 1985 was clearly not as restrictive. And national officers of the Red Cross made clear they would not remove the older products from the shelves. Deliveries of the questionable material kept coming until April to the national headquarters, as late as June in at least one centre, and these were added to the inventory. The Red Cross insists that it lived up to the distribution target dates set at the consensus meeting in December 1984. But some hospitals, at least, used contaminated unheated products even after July 1.

This reluctance to part with those now-risky blood products appears to have been partly due to the cost of the replacements. C. A. Anhorn, the Red Cross operations manager for blood product services, had prepared cost estimates for the December consensus meeting. He noted that replacement of non-heated concentrates by the new version would cost $1 million to $1.3 million a year more. If the transition did not go smoothly, the cost could be $1.5 million to $2 million higher. "This represents an annual increase of from

19 to 25 per cent in the cost of providing AHF concentrate for hemophilia care in Canada," Anhorn reported.

Spot purchases of heat-treated products, which might have helped some hemophiliacs through the crisis period, were even more costly. Contracted supplies would add two cents to the eleven cents per AHF unit cost. Buying on the spot market would mean additional costs of five cents a unit.

Today's Red Cross officials, who are in the unenviable position of having to clean up after the elephant, claim the organization acted expeditiously to shift over to heat-treated products. Stephen Vick says that as soon as the Bureau of Biologics issued its November 16, 1984, directive, the Red Cross withdrew an order for non-heated supplies for the coming year. Cutter was notified and asked if it could handle extra plasma diverted on November 20 from Connaught, which had no heat-treatment capability. The U.S. firm was also asked to start making heat-treated product immediately.

"This was before we had approval from the funding agency, the Canadian Blood Committee," says Vick. "We needed approval from the CBC to introduce heat-treated products. We were at a standstill as far as buying for 1985 and that's why we wanted the CBC to make a quick decision because we wanted to get our orders into place. . . . Within a few days all of these events took place." The approval came December 11. The Red Cross, Vick says, had already met with suppliers to ascertain product availability.

On December 14, 1984, the Red Cross issued a request to blood fractionators for a year's supply of 40 million units of heat-treated products. The firms were asked to respond by January 4, 1985, with samples to be provided a week later. The suppliers were to disclose the source of the blood, provide evidence of steps to exclude donors at high risk for AIDS, and give documented proof the products were treated to inactivate viruses, including hepatitis and HIV. The products were to be delivered the first week of each month, starting April 1, 1985, when 10 million units were due. During April, the Red

Cross also expected to receive another 3.7 million units derived from the Canadian plasma shipped south to Cutter for processing.

Meanwhile, Baxter-Hyland had submitted an offer in December, its second since November 1983, to supply heat-treated product to the Red Cross. The company also offered to pass along its heat-processing technology, royalty-free. The Red Cross simply relayed the technology offer to Connaught, the only significant Canadian-based fractionator. The offer by Baxter may have been altruistic or, more likely in the cutthroat fractionation business, in the hope of getting a share in a highly competitive market. Whatever the case, Baxter was left the unwanted suitor.

On January 31, the Red Cross issued its orders. Clearly, the Bureau of Biologics' initial hope of delivery in mid-January or mid-February was out the window. Cutter was to supply 30 million units, and 10 million units were to come from Armour, whose heat-treated product was not even licensed in Canada at the time. The Bureau said there was no problem — Armour could be licensed by February. The contract was split between two companies "to diffuse any negative impact of the U.S. market situation on supplies of Factor VIII in Canada."

A question that perplexes and angers many hemophiliacs today is why the Red Cross did not take advantage of Baxter's offer to supply heat-treated products. A Red Cross "excuse sheet" issued in July 1993 sets out four reasons. All are disputable.

First, the Red Cross argues, the Baxter process was licensed to kill hepatitis B, not HIV. This is a curious argument, because product monographs attached to the Cutter licence issued in November 1984 and Armour's of April 1985 show that both referred to inactivation of hepatitis, and only mention HIV in passing as a potential danger.

The key study demonstrating that heat treatment killed retroviruses had indeed been conducted in Cutter's California labs. The findings had been widely hailed as the development that could rid blood products of the HIV scourge. There was evidently hope in Ottawa that heat treatment was the solution, but authorities naturally wanted to be sure that it would not adversely affect the product. As pressure mounted for the use of heat-purified products, the Cutter request for licensing, initially made in July 1984, had been quickly advanced for regulatory approval. Heartening words had been murmured by Red Cross experts about Cutter, a favoured partner with a longstanding cosy relationship.

Cutter had obtained a Canadian licence for its heat-treated product on November 13, 1984. Three days later the Bureau of Biologics called for the switch-over to heat-treated products as soon as feasible. But Cutter's product monograph makes it clear that hepatitis, not AIDS, was the primary target. "Koate-HT has undergone a heating step in an attempt to reduce the risk of transmission of hepatitis and other infectious diseases," it states under "Clinical Pharmacology." A second section, entitled "Warnings," notes the high risk of hepatitis with the use of clotting factors. There's only one reference to AIDS in the seven-page document: "Isolated cases of acquired immune deficiency syndrome have been reported in hemophiliacs who have received blood and/or coagulation factor concentrates, including Factor VIII concentrates. It is not known if the disease is due to a transmitted specific agent, secondary to multiple antigenic exposures, or to some other mechanisms. The physician and patient should consider that Factor VIII concentrates may be associated with the transmission of AIDS and weigh the benefits of therapy accordingly." There is no claim that the new heat-purified Cutter product is effective against AIDS transmission.

So why did Canadian users of clotting concentrates have to wait for adequate supplies of the Cutter product? Why did the Red Cross not place an order for an interim supply of Baxter's product when Cutter's more intensely treated product was in short supply? Couldn't Baxter's have been used as a bridge until adequate amounts of Cutter's product were available? Vick says he has seen no evidence that this was a significant option, because Baxter was unable to guarantee supply. Baxter officials, for their part, decline to supply numbers on what they might have had available.

Durhane Wong-Rieger, the CHS president as of May 1994, says

both the Bureau and the Red Cross claim they sent Canadian-source plasma into the United States to Cutter because it was the only licensed heat-treating process for Canada. "That is not true. Unless they had forgotten that they had already licensed Baxter, which I don't think is really likely, they were setting forth a deliberate misconception." Wong-Rieger says CHS representatives checked to see if the Cutter product had been licensed as effective against HIV while the Baxter licence was granted as an anti-hepatitis product. "Not true. Cutter put in their request for licensing well before they had been able to prove that it was effective against HTLV-III. So their application was exactly the same as Baxter's. It was really for hepatitis B."

Armour Pharmaceuticals had also applied for approval of a dry heat-treated concentrate in the fall of 1984. Again, the specific target of that product was hepatitis, especially the variety known as non-A, non-B (later called hepatitis C). The Health Department did not issue a notice of compliance that would allow use of the product in Canada until April 12, 1985.

In any case, a blind eye is sometimes turned to licences. In recent times, unlicensed Factor IX concentrates have been used widely in Canada, and routinely obtained through emergency drug release.

The second reason given by the Red Cross for the rejection of Baxter's product was that it would take the Bureau of Biologics "several months" to license Baxter's method for deactivating HIV. As it happened, the Bureau failed to keep its promised deadline for licensing Armour and the mid-April approval came two weeks after the first deliveries were due. In any case, Baxter's product had already been licensed for Canadian use and HIV was a much more easily destroyed virus than hepatitis B.

Third, the Red Cross pointed out that the Baxter heat-treating method differed from that set out in the November 16 Bureau of Biologics directive. In fact, it turned out to be safer than the Armour product. Although Baxter's virus-killing method was not as "robust" as Cutter's, the dry-heated Armour product which was acceptable to the Red Cross was later implicated in HIV infections that occurred in 1987, well after concentrates were believed safe against the virus. Baxter's dry-heat process was at the same temperature as Armour's (60 degrees Celsius) and 72 hours long, more than twice that of Armour's.

William Mutert, Baxter's current vice-president of global marketing, agrees the Baxter Hemofil-T was not as good as had been hoped in neutralizing its initial target, hepatitis B. "Unfortunately, it did not neutralize that virus, but it was effective against HIV, a more heat-labile virus." In other words, it would have done the job.

Finally, the Red Cross argues Baxter could not guarantee delivery of its product on "short notice." The reality is that neither of the two companies chosen delivered on time. It took Cutter and Armour a minimum of five and a half months to deliver after the consensus conference, and the bulk of the ordered supplies arrived closer to seven months later. If Baxter had such problems making deliveries, why did they rush in with offers to supply the product? And according to the Red Cross's own chronology, their preferred supplier, Cutter, ended up begging for a delay in delivery until the end of June.

Vick says Baxter had some supply in the United States. "We asked them to bid on it, and they bid on smaller quantities. But they weren't prepared to guarantee delivery to the levels that we required. Armour and Cutter did guarantee delivery by April," he adds. "When you're negotiating a contract, you go with the people who say they can dance rather than with people who say they can't." But both chosen suppliers missed their "guaranteed" delivery dates. What if would-be dancers tell their partners they can foxtrot, and turn out to be fumble-footed?

By March 11, 1985, Cutter was pleading for an extension, according to the Red Cross chronology. It could not honour the contracted delivery schedule because of serious depletion of inventories due to overselling of production and "poor inventory management." How would the end of June do for the first deliveries? Not acceptable, the Red Cross retorted.

Meanwhile, Armour was still having trouble getting a licence.

Four of thirteen lots submitted by the company for testing had proven inadequate. The only product the Red Cross was "guaranteed" was the Cutter-processed Canadian plasma. That fell through, too; the Canadian-source product didn't arrive until June.

Armour was finally licensed in mid-April, two months late. On April 25, about 1.6 million Armour units rolled into the Red Cross. Then the first Cutter product, 2.5 million units, arrived April 29. On May 1, another Armour shipment arrived, bringing the total Red Cross heat-treated inventory to 7.8 million units. But the deliveries were a month late and 10 million units short.

One might have thought that given the breakdowns in delivery and the Red Cross's proclaimed determination to obtain products as quickly as possible, they might have turned elsewhere. But they stood by their chosen, struggling suppliers and have maintained that there were no viable alternatives.

Much debate has centred on the issue of how much supply was available at the time. A Red Cross position paper prepared in September 1985 said deliveries did not meet the plan before July 8 "because of worldwide scarcities in the supply of heat-treated product." That position is maintained today by Vick, who adds that manufacturers were still trying to get licensed. "Everybody was scrambling to get it."

"Many companies were overselling products and were unable to meet their delivery deadlines," goes the Red Cross explanation. This was certainly true; two of the chief culprits were Cutter and Armour — the firms the Red Cross had selected as its suppliers.

But court testimony during France's tainted blood trials indicates there were six European companies with significant quantities of heat-treated products at that time. What efforts were made to obtain supplies there?

Supplies were definitely available before the fall of 1984. But once the news spread from the United States, many users wanted to switch to the heated products. "At that point, I imagine it would be more a case of being first in line, making sure you were in line," says David Page.

Jack Reasor is president of the Market Research Bureau in Laguna Beach, California, a firm that has been doing market reports on plasma products for twenty years. In a February 1994 interview, he chuckled when told the Canadian Red Cross maintains there was no heat-treated blood product available for export to Canada at the end of 1984 and early 1985.

"Who says there wasn't!" Reasor exclaimed. "There were at least a dozen fractionators around the world who had product."

Another authority is Tom Drees, now a private consultant but in the early 1980s the president of Alpha Therapeutics, a producer of Factor VIII and Factor IX concentrates.

Heat-treated products were approved in the U.S. for Baxter in early 1983, for Alpha in January 1984, and for Cutter in February 1984, Drees pointed out in a February 1994 interview.

"There was plenty of material available," he said from Pasadena, California. "I think the problem was that the Canadian Red Cross simply had not budgeted for the increase in price that was required when the heat treatment came in, because the heat treatment caused a yield loss of 40 to 60 per cent, which had to be made up for in an increase in cost. I suspect, although I don't know this for sure, they simply didn't want to pay the higher price."

Drees said the Red Cross had maintained they couldn't get a confirmed delivery promise. "My reply to that is, if you are a businessman and you want to get a confirmed delivery promise, you place an order. It sounds to me like they were dancing around and saying, 'Well, can you deliver it if I place an order?' and the answer to that is, 'Place an order, and that's how you know you are going to get it.'

"This is not unique to the Canadian Red Cross," Drees said. "This is typical of all the blood people at this period of time, who were dancing around and playing games, putting their heads in the sand. They were afraid that if they faced up to it, people would say, 'Gee, maybe there's something wrong with that stuff!' And sure enough, there was something wrong with that stuff."

After Drees appeared in a CBC news special on February 14, 1994,

Vick responded for the Red Cross that Alpha Therapeutics had not been licensed by the Bureau of Biologics to sell heat-treated concentrate at that time.

"I wasn't making that statement based on Alpha," replies Drees. "I was making that statement based on the whole industry. I had left Alpha in 1983, but I was very conversant with what was going on in the industry."

Vick grins when asked about his disagreement with Drees. "I don't want to cast aspersions, but talk to some of the other people in the industry about Tom. He has been accused of having a selective memory."

Vick says the message that may come out is, Yes there was product available, but it was being allocated. As product became available, rather than sell to one client or one group of clients, companies would share it among their customer base. He notes that all the suppliers for Canada at the time were American. While Vick wasn't involved in the 1984–85 situation, he refers to a later experience he dealt with personally in 1987. "When shortages occur, there is a lot of pressure on U.S. companies to meet the U.S. requirements first."

Bill Mindell believes there might be something to the Red Cross argument that supplies were not available. "The standard of care changed overnight. So, why in the world would they think Canada is the only country looking for this stuff? I can't understand how it would be available all that fast. On the other hand, if all we had to do was pay more money, then maybe we should have paid more money."

Mindell speculates that those who attended the 1984 consensus conference may have known that large numbers of hemophiliacs were already infected. They may have taken a position that the damage was done. "I don't know whether that's an ethical stand. I don't know if that entered into the decision at all."

Even if we believe that the Red Cross was trying to obtain supplies "quickly," it was less than swift in doling them out once they were received. Of the available inventory of heat-treated units in May

1985, only a tiny portion of the supply was distributed to consumers during that month. The rest was held back. Meanwhile, leaders of the Hemophilia Society were urging distribution of the product on hand. When the advisory sub-committee to the Canadian Blood Committee met April 15, the Red Cross said the forty million ordered units would be distributed over a twelve-month period. Ken Poyser asked why supplies weren't to be immediately given out. The available quantity was sufficient to meet current needs, Poyser argued. Instead, Roger Perrault restated the consensus conference decision to begin distribution on May 1, 1985, with a two-month transition period. The Hemophilia Society had interpreted the proposal approved by the conference as calling for distribution as soon as feasible, "before May," with an eight-week transition period thereafter. According to this view, May was the latest allowable starting date, not the confirmed date for the launch.

The Red Cross thought otherwise. "This, in the Red Cross's opinion, given the state of supply known at the time, would not have been a responsible decision, as to effect a full conversion, without an assurance of an ability to maintain a supply thereafter, would defeat the purpose of the conversion," says a 1993 Red Cross press release on the implementation of heat-treated product.

It was an arbitrary decision at a critical time that may have cost many lives. When heat-treated product was ordered and the implementation plan drawn up, the HIV-infection rate among severe hemophiliacs was believed to be about 55 per cent. When the final toll came in, the rate was closer to 80 per cent. It's questionable whether stockpiling can be justified. By May 15, Cutter had confirmed it was going to make its June commitments. At that point, the Red Cross had enough supply on hand to make a full conversion. Instead, its bureaucrats chose to hold on until the products had arrived on site.

There were other alternatives available. The Red Cross could have issued a portion of the supply with a strict warning that use should be limited, or supplemented with available cryoprecipitate. Hemophiliacs were accustomed to frequent supply shortages and could have adjusted. Furthermore, many of them for years had used cryo at home and concentrates when they were travelling.

Vick was asked if that option was considered. "Well, the process that was followed, I think, was the right process," he says.

How hard did Red Cross officials try to obtain backup or bridging supplies from companies like Baxter? Baxter seemed only too eager to deal and had offered to supply smaller quantities than the Red Cross wanted in its contract. If the issue was safety, says Lindee David, the CHS executive director in June 1994, they should have purchased whatever supplies were available.

On March 7, 1985, results from Canada's National Advisory Committee on AIDS (NAC-AIDS) reaffirmed there was a high probability of contamination among hemophiliacs. The same month similar results were released by the National Hemophilia Foundation in the United States. A majority of American hemophiliacs tested HIV-antibody-positive but "the medical significance of a positive test is unknown in terms of its predictive value," the Foundation said.

Dr. Naylor, director of blood products and services for the Red Cross, issued a detailed memo on March 20, 1985, to Blood Transfusion Service medical directors, setting out the agency game plan for distribution of heat-treated products. Naylor told them that forty million units had been ordered, and that between May 1 and July 1 "limited amounts" would be distributed to the blood transfusion centres. "The greater proportion of coagulation factor products will continue to be supplied in non-heated form during this transition period," Naylor wrote.

"After July 1, heat-treated coagulation factor products will be made exclusively available and non-heat-treated products will no longer be distributed," Naylor continued. "During the transition period May 1 to July 1, all centres will receive small amounts of heat-treated Factor VIII and Factor IX that will be a proportion of their normal monthly utilization; this proportion will be determined according to the estimated number of patients that are eligible to receive heat-treated products preferentially according to the criteria that will be established at the April 19 meeting of the Canadian Hemophilia Society's medical and scientific advisory committee (MSAC).

"The majority of hemophilia patients that have been on long-term concentrate therapy will continue to be supplied with non-heat-treated products until after July 1."

Naylor said he anticipated that priority for heat-treated products would be given to young hemophiliacs who used cryoprecipitate, and to mild hemophiliacs who used coagulants infrequently in recent years.

The significance of this should not be underestimated. The job of deciding which hemophiliacs should get priority in the distribution of the new heat-treated concentrates had been given to the MSAC. But Naylor's memo revealed preconceived ideas about who should receive the product. By jumping the gun and issuing his own marching orders early, Naylor was usurping MSAC's role. He had made assumptions about infection among long-term users of concentrates, and ensured a conservative distribution of the heat-treated products. His assumptions would carry a lot of weight among Red Cross regional directors.

On April 26, Naylor received the MSAC recommendations. These were to be implemented "at once," said the attached letter from Dr. Robert Card, the MSAC chair. As Naylor expected, the heat-treated products were to go first to previously untreated or rarely treated hemophiliacs who might need them during the conversion period, to young children, and to those who normally used cryoprecipitate but might require concentrates for travel. The distribution was to be done equitably across Canada and decisions as to who got priority were to be made by hemophilia clinic directors after consultation with the Red Cross.

But a significant group, listed second by Card, seems to have been ignored. Indeed, it was left out of the instructions Naylor had issued in March. "Previously treated patients known to be sero-negative for HTLV-III antibodies" were also supposed to receive the new products. There seems to have been no direction given by Naylor or others in the Red Cross to give these uninfected hemophiliacs any priority.

In a second memo on April 29, Naylor reinforced his directive about limited distribution and his recommendation that the majority of hemophiliacs not receive the new products until July 1. It was the day the first Cutter concentrates arrived.

Roger Perrault reviewed the Red Cross distribution plan at a National Advisory Committee on AIDS meeting on May 15. He said that there was an "understanding" at hemophilia treatment centres that "current inventories were to be used first." The implication was the Red Cross intended to use the risky non-heated concentrates regardless of the availability of the new heat-processed products. Given Canada's increasing dependence on U.S.–source concentrates and Perrault's remark at the same session that high-risk donors in the United States were still donating blood, the level of responsibility seemed to be low.

On May 30, Naylor's memo machine was at work again. "Routine centre requirements were to be met with untreated products." Naylor said there was an insufficient supply of the heat-treated products to fill all routine requests. The strict distribution would mean that physicians would have to pick and choose, and make explicit requests for the new products. This prioritization led to "heart-wrenching" decisions for doctors, one regional director told the Krever inquiry. The most severe cases of hemophilia — those patients who required product every week or every month (in some cases almost daily) — would continue to receive the largest amounts of the riskiest products. Milder hemophiliacs, who rarely required infusions, got the new, safer products. Why the stinginess? The answer seems to be that the Red Cross, and Naylor in particular, was determined to use up all the non-treated products in the pipeline.

At a time of acute danger, therefore, the prime agency responsible for Canada's blood supply responded sluggishly in distributing the new, safer concentrates. May 1, 1985, had been cited by Perrault as the "latest" date to start the transition to heat-treated products. Despite the supply delays, the Red Cross national office had about 25,000 vials of Factor VIII concentrates on hand by that date, sufficient for a two-month supply for all Canadian hemophiliacs. Yet the Red Cross's own figures reveal that fewer than 1,200 vials were distributed that month. By June 3, there were about 50,000 vials on the shelves — enough for four months — but fewer than 4,500 had been handed out. A similar pattern held for Factor IX concentrates. Meanwhile, between January and June about 53,000 vials of non-heat-treated factor had been distributed. Only 6,000 returned in the subsequent recall.

The hold-back of the new product was deliberate. In a report dated September 27, 1985, C. A. Anhorn of the Red Cross said the Blood Transfusion Service "planned to re-establish its operating inventory prior to implementation" of the consensus conference decision.

The Winnipeg Red Cross centre seems to have been extraordinarily tight-fisted with the heat-treated products it had on hand. As early as March 1985, the Winnipeg Red Cross regional director, Dr. Marlis Schroeder, was warning hemophiliacs not to expect too much too soon. She told them at a meeting to expect a "very slow switch-over" to the new concentrates, probably spread over three months. "I would be very surprised if it [the completion date] was July 1." Her prediction was that by fall all of the products distributed would be heat-treated.

The first load of heat-treated products started arriving in Winnipeg on April 30, but despite demand from hemophiliacs only a minuscule amount was handed out over the next two months. The first load that arrived was 130 vials. No more arrived in May, and none was distributed. The last delivery of 110 vials of non-heated products came on June 4. Another 225 heat-treated vials rolled in on June 12 and 290 more on June 25. By the end of June, a total of 645 heat-treated vials had been delivered.

Very little was issued. Four vials for children in rural Manitoba were distributed on June 8 and again on June 20. And on June 30, seven more were picked up by an adult Winnipeg hemophiliac, Ed Kubin. That was a total of 15 of the 645 vials available — a little more than 2 per cent of the heat-treated inventory. Meanwhile, about

450 untreated vials were distributed over that same period and at least 100 were used by hemophiliacs, the rest returned when the recall went out in July. These numbers suggest that the available supplies of heat-treated products would have been enough to meet the needs.

Schroeder was asked at the Krever inquiry why distribution didn't begin earlier. There was concern, she told commission lawyer Marlys Edwardh, that if a child required major surgery, there wouldn't be enough heat-treated product to provide for them. But why couldn't some of the supply have been held back to cover such eventualities, and the rest distributed?

CHS lawyer Bonnie Tough pointed out that many hemophiliacs had understood the Red Cross would not issue the heat-treated products until old inventories had been used up. That notion came from a videotaped meeting in March 1985 in which Schroeder warned hemophiliacs not to stockpile large supplies of non-heat-treated products at home because they would not be accepted if they were taken back to the centre. The intent, Schroeder replied, was for hemophiliacs to use products on hand "down to the minimum" before heat-treated supplies would be provided.

Schroeder, apparently trying to justify the late distribution, also told Tough there were doubts at the time about the effectiveness of heat treatment in inactivating HIV. Yet, in mid-August a national office memo directed that "all untested plasma" should be shipped to fractionators before November 30, 1985. Why, if there was uncertainty about heat treatment, would unscreened plasma be sent to make blood products? Tough asked. There was a strong feeling the process did, in fact, work, Schroeder replied, apparently contradicting herself.

The Winnipeg centre was not alone. The Nova Scotia and New Brunswick Red Cross divisions failed hemophiliacs, too. The provincial director in New Brunswick, which has the highest rate of HIV infection among hemophiliacs among the provinces, was not about to challenge the priorities sent him by the Red Cross national headquarters in 1985, in spite of his misgivings. John MacKay said he thought he could be fired if he disobeyed the guidelines. It was not his job to exercise independent thought. The result was that four vials of possibly contaminated factor were distributed on June 30 when nearly 850 heat-treated vials were available for hemophiliacs the next day.

Nova Scotia's Red Cross followed a similar pattern. In June, while 165 units of heat-treated material sat on the shelves awaiting distribution on July 1, nearly 70 possibly-contaminated units were sent out. These decisions show the Red Cross authorities in those provinces chose the most conservative option available to them, rather than acting to protect the users of blood.

There was a profound reluctance, too, to distribute the new products from the Hamilton, Ontario, Red Cross centre. In mid-May, a memo was sent to blood bank directors at the region's twenty-eight hospitals. "Until the available supplies of non-heat-treated clotting factor concentrates are used, the heat-treated products will be reserved exclusively for the treatment of those patients that fulfill the criteria" of the MSAC. The memo made no reference to the completion of the transition by July 1. During May, at a meeting of hemophilia specialists and the Red Cross, the July 1 date was mentioned but it was stated that "it was important all other Factor VIII should be used up before using the heat-treated."

Meanwhile, the heat-processed concentrates were piling up at the Hamilton centre. The first allotment, 115 vials, arrived on April 30. By the beginning of June, the inventory was 862 heat-treated vials and only 251 non-treated. By mid-June, hospitals were starting to ship back non-heat-treated product, but astonishingly, some of these were re-issued as late as June 28. By the end of June, the Hamilton centre had a heat-treated inventory of 1,459 vials, but none of the old product.

Dr. Morris Blajchman, the centre's director at the time, was asked at the Krever inquiry in October 1994 why, in the face of a "fairly extensive" inventory of heat-treated factor, the Red Cross would have re-issued the hazardous material.

"My recollection is that I did not take care in the centre to instruct them not to re-issue returns," Blajchman replied. He added that there was "no evidence available at that time" that heat treatment would prevent the transmission of AIDS. The inserts in the boxes of Factor VIII "only referred to hepatitis."

In a testy exchange with lawyer Ken Arenson, Blajchman defended himself by saying it would have been irresponsible for him to distribute the heat-treated product to hemophiliacs not included on the MSAC list, only to find that there would be none available to someone who was covered. "I am not a prophet. Neither are you," Blajchman replied. "If I were a prophet, I would have done things differently."

In Newfoundland, the manager of the Red Cross transfusion service broke with instructions from the national headquarters and, without the knowledge of his medical director, turned over heat-treated products to the province's hemophilia centre for distribution.

Newfoundland was the only province east of Quebec where some of the new concentrates were distributed in May 1985. The Red Cross medical director, Richard Huntsman, told the Krever inquiry in August 1994 that he had only learned four weeks earlier of the initiative that his staff member, Tom Peddle, had undertaken nearly a decade ago.

Peddle had told him that as the new products arrived, he sent them out to the treaters, with the exception of a few vials held back for emergency. "I felt like dropping on my knees to say thank you!" exclaimed Huntsman. "He in fact did what should have been done. He said to the treaters: 'This is your problem. It's not mine.'"

Huntsman admitted he would not have acted as swiftly as his colleague. "I was under the impression right up to late June that this product was in desperately short supply. Therefore, I would have been much more tempted to have followed the protocol up to 11:59 p.m. on June 30. That was the message handed down.

"As it turned out, I thanked him for disobeying a string of instructions."

Picture yourself as the director of a regional blood bank in the spring of 1985. You receive an order from a senior national officer of the Red Cross saying some heat-treated concentrates will be distributed to your region but they will be in short supply. The directive sets out a procedure for distribution of the blood products. These instructions are reinforced in further memos. He omits the second group listed by the MSAC as eligible for heat-treated products — patients who have used concentrates but are known to have, thus far, dodged the virus. Then, he tells his regional officers in charge of blood-products distribution to supply non-heated concentrates to fill "routine" requests.

What we see is a conservative pattern of distribution that seems to have taken no account of an urgent situation. And that choice was not necessary. For those not yet infected in the early summer of 1985, it was in many cases a death sentence.

Chapter 6

OPTIONS DISMISSED

"I believe there are lives, and the quality of lives, at stake here.
If the policies and recommendations I have been pushing
are incorrect, we gain or lose nothing. If the present policies
of the [Red Cross] are incorrect, we lose everything."
BILL MINDELL, FORMER CHAIR OF HEMOPHILIA
ONTARIO'S FACTOR PRODUCTS COMMITTEE, JULY 1985

Those who foresaw in the early 1980s that HIV and AIDS could be transmitted through the blood concentrates used by hemophiliacs were also the first to look for alternatives. The increasingly questionable dried products were no doubt convenient. They were effective in halting bleeds. They weren't nearly as messy as older clotting agents. But many people believed if there was risk of major contamination, they had to be avoided. For those standing in the path of a runaway freight train, a step backward might be the only way.

As early as January 1983, a working group of virologists and immunologists for the Canadian Red Cross suggested blood banks should prepare to deal with an increased demand for the older blood product, cryoprecipitate. "Altered T-lymphocyte function, a component of AIDS, has been reported to be less frequent in hemophilia patients who are treated with cryoprecipitate, rather than anti-hemophilic factor concentrates," they reported in a memo to medical directors. "Although this does not necessarily imply that cryoprecipitate is free of risk, this finding may lead to an increased demand for cryoprecipitate."

Even those who most feared the spread of AIDS through blood likely did not appreciate how immense the danger was at the time, but some specialists in both Canada and the United States had guessed that exposure of their patients to the smallest number of donors possible was the best route to take. In the manufacture of concentrates, the plasma from thousands of donors was pooled. With cryoprecipitate, a single donor's plasma could be used to produce one bag. Depending upon size, body weight, and severity of bleed, a hemophiliac might pool four to twelve bags in a single injection. In theory, that meant reduced risk of a user being infected by a contaminated donor.

Medical advisors to both the National Hemophilia Foundation in the United States and the Canadian Hemophilia Society also suggested cryoprecipitate was safer, and the advice was taken to heart in some circles. Use of the old standby rose in Canada in 1983 and 1984. In some cases, younger children had not been switched to the concentrates, and when fears arose about transmission of the AIDS virus through blood, their doctors decided to keep their young patients on what they believed to be the tried and true product and wait for developments.

Cryoprecipitate, also used in heart surgery as well as hemophilia, had been a lifesaver when it first appeared, and was destined to be again. The product, which was processed at Red Cross regional centres, had power to stop bleeding that was many times greater than whole plasma. But it was an inconvenient and time-consuming remedy. There could be all manner of extraneous material in the sticky fluid. Some bags had a pinkish hue from unseparated red blood cells. The risk of reactions was high. And there were "duds," in which the active ingredient failed to work. Moreover, cryo had to be kept frozen until use. Hemophiliacs who travelled sometimes carried large foam cartons packed with dry ice inside cardboard boxes. When needed, cryo had to be thawed in lukewarm water. It was then mixed with saline solution in an intravenous apparatus, which was hung from a hook or a stand, and dripped into the veins through a butterfly needle, usually inserted at the elbow or hand. An alternative would be to mix the cryoprecipitate and saline and use a large syringe to slowly inject the clotting factor. This was faster than the drip method but was frowned upon by some doctors and hemophiliacs, too, who feared it might "blow" a vein or overwhelm the circulatory system. Home users needed to make sure they had the bags of saline, a supply of the intravenous apparatuses, bags of cryo, butterfly needles, alcohol swabs, a rubber tourniquet to tie around the arm to make veins stand out for easier puncture, and sterilized pads. Travellers carrying boxes stamped "Human Blood Products" on a plane or train, or stuffing them in the baggage compartment of a bus, could expect perplexed stares from fellow passengers.

As the newer and less bulky concentrates became more commonly available, the use of cryoprecipitate in Canada had fallen to a low of 141,000 units a year in 1982, down from the peak of 363,000 units in 1978. But in 1983, the trend reversed and 164,000 units of cryo were used. In 1984, that rose to 192,000 units. Some doctors were clearly alert to the greater degree of safety inherent in cryoprecipitate. "There was some shift back to an alternate method of treatment," Dr. Roger Perrault, Red Cross national director of blood services between 1974 and 1986, told the parliamentary subcommittee early in 1993.

As more treating doctors and hemophiliacs became aware of the risk in the non-heat-treated products, their use declined. Red Cross figures compiled in the fall of 1985 show that after the December 1984 consensus conference, the volume of Factor VIII issued fell by 16 per cent. Once new heat-treated products were fully distributed in July 1985, the volume issued soared by 61 per cent.

Logic suggested cryo was safer than concentrates. Although cryo could harbour HIV, too, with a smaller number of contributors, the chance the supply would be contaminated was far less. In some areas or hospitals, cryoprecipitate was again the treatment of choice.

Dr. Annette Poon, who runs the blood bank at Toronto's Hospital for Sick Children, says in 1982 or 1983 efforts were made to avoid potentially dangerous American-source concentrates. She described a three-step process. "In the early years [of the AIDS scare], we switched from concentrate. When there was a suspicion of HIV being transmitted by concentrate, we switched as many as possible back to cryoprecipitate," she told the Krever inquiry in March 1994.

Some children had reactions to cryo and others who needed significant surgery required concentrates. "In those situations, the next step after cryoprecipitate would be the Canadian product, Connaught Factor VIII, because at the time we felt the risk of HIV transmission was less than with the product coming from the United States. We seldom used the product from the States, unless we were actually out of the Canadian product completely." When that did occur, the blood bank notified the hematologist, who would decide whether an operation should proceed or whether it could be delayed until Canadian concentrates or cryo was available. That policy continued until the heat-treated concentrates arrived in mid-1985.

A record kept for an eleven-year-old Toronto hemophiliac for a two-month period in late 1982 shows a mix of products being used. In that time, the boy had seven separate bleeding episodes requiring more than one injection. Three were treated solely by cryo, one was handled with a mix of cryo and Canadian-made Connaught concentrate, two were dealt with by an American-source product, and in one Connaught only was used. This was a fairly typical pattern.

In Calgary, a succession of doctors were on the scene in the early 1980s who believed cryoprecipitate was a safer choice than the new-fangled concentrates. Dr. Tom Bowen, Red Cross medical director for the Calgary centre from 1981–85, was concerned about transmission of an infectious agent through blood. Bowen, who says he was always "fairly vocal" about the advantages of his preferred product, told a group of Calgary hemophiliac families in April 1983 that cryoprecipitate was likely safer.

In July 1983, he wrote a memo to the Red Cross national office suggesting all recipients of blood products should be exposed to "a minimum number of donations." Cryo from a single donor would be safer than concentrate that might be made from one thousand to two thousand, Bowen argued.

Bowen told the Krever hearings that his predecessor, Dr. Andrew Kaegi, had encouraged Calgary hemophiliacs to remain on the older coagulant. That stance was reinforced by Dr. Man-Chiu Poon, the newly arrived hemophilia clinic director in 1983. Poon made a conscious effort to keep the younger children on cryoprecipitate as long as possible. There was no scientific proof that cryo was safer, Bowen said. It was just a "gut feeling."

The choice for Calgary proved to be right. The HIV-infection rate among Alberta's hemophiliacs is one of the lowest in the country, and Calgary's is about one-fourth of the rate in the province's other major city, Edmonton.

In his appearance before Krever, the long-haired, white-bearded Bowen both sounded and looked like a guru. There were two different gut feelings, he noted, one for cryoprecipitate and one for concentrate. Most national Red Cross officials, for example, believed concentrates were safer because of dilution of potential contaminants and the greater degree of processing. "One gets to looking like a fool in the end perhaps, and it looks like they might know something. But neither knew any more than the other. They had the same crystal balls. They just had different pictures coming out of them."

At the time, some doctors were apparently being told that cryoprecipitate, less convenient but safer, was in scarce supply. Today, there seems little evidence to bear that out. Before the parliamentary subcommittee on health issues on February 25, 1993, Roger Perrault twice affirmed cryo use as a viable alternative to concentrates. It was available. That is also confirmed by Stephen Vick, the current Red Cross national director for manufacturing, who says today there was no shortage of cryo at any time. Vick added, however, that hemophiliacs didn't want to switch back to the less convenient product.

That presumes, of course, that they knew there was a choice. Few hemophiliacs recall ever being told by their doctors that cryo was likely safer than concentrates. James Kreppner, for example, says if someone had informed him of the peril he would have gone back to cryoprecipitate. The Toronto lawyer says he had two relatives who stayed with the older coagulant just because they had a conservative streak and were used to it. "I thought they were foolish not to move with the times," Kreppner told the Krever inquiry. Today, Kreppner is HIV-positive. His relatives are both negative.

In his parliamentary testimony, Dr. Roger Perrault was asked what option there would have been if all Factor VIII had been held back. "One of the alternatives would have been to convert the whole system to cryo." Indeed, production of cryoprecipitate from plasma was actually more efficient than dried-concentrate production.

"The efficiency of the Factor VIII concentrate manufacture was 20 per cent to 30 per cent," Perrault commented. "In other words, from 1,000 units in a litre of plasma you could extract by this difficult process 200 to 300 units of Factor VIII. In the cryoprecipitate, it was 50 per cent to 60 per cent efficient, and sometimes you could do it almost to 70 per cent.

"Had the system — and we're theorizing — converted to cryo, and that would have been extremely inconvenient for the hemophiliacs and we have to take that into account, we could probably have been nationally self-sufficient."

But Perrault absolved the Red Cross of any role in making that choice. "Those were not Red Cross decisions, those were treating decisions." He was saying that doctors and hospitals could have chosen what materials their patients should use.

In his parliamentary testimony, Perrault had admitted that supplies of a safer alternative were available at the time. When some hemophiliacs and treating doctors lobbied for the removal of non-heat-treated concentrates in the early to mid-eighties, they had been told there was no alternative but to continue using the risky products. Hemophiliacs would die if they did not treat, they were told.

If Perrault knew that there were sufficient supplies of cryoprecipitate to make a switch, at least some of his underlings at the Red Cross, and apparently some hematologists, did not. The regional picture, however, does not seem to be consistent.

In early 1983, significant increases in cryoprecipitate use were reported in the Toronto and Hamilton areas. Indeed, John Derrick of the Red Cross noted that if the trend continued, "immense revenues may be lost by the fractionators." Those companies had invested millions of dollars into the production of the now-suspect concentrates. If the switch back to cryo continued, it could lead to increased costs for other products, he added, as the manufacturers tried to offset their losses. "This will not, however, be a consideration in taking precautionary steps, should they be necessary," Derrick added.

Dr. Noel Buskard, Red Cross medical director for British Columbia at the time, expected use of cryoprecipitate to rise in his region and alerted hospital blood bankers to be prepared for increased demand. To his surprise, however, there was no significant rise.

Bowen says there was always a good deal of cryoprecipitate available in Alberta, and his centre could have geared up to produce more. "We were prepared as a donor centre to provide whatever cryoprecipitate was being requested." Saskatchewan, too, had sufficient amounts.

Marlis Schroeder, medical director at the Winnipeg centre, was asked at a gathering of hemophiliacs in March 1985 whether they should change from concentrates to cryoprecipitate until heat-treated products were available.

"If we're going to switch over completely, we would basically have to double production of cryoprecipitate, and that is logistically impossible," she said. The Red Cross would need more staff and more money, and would have trouble quick-freezing plasma collected from cities far away from the regional centre. "We will try to provide as much cryo as we can. We will require advance notice and we will tell you whether or not we can provide you with that product because of the logistical problems."

At the Krever inquiry in June 1994, Schroeder seemed surprised that with hemophiliacs increasingly nervous about blood, there had been no requests for cryo. "We would have been able to switch to cryoprecipitate to a greater extent than was done, but no one requested it." Schroeder also agreed there would have been no supply problem if severe hemophiliacs had switched over for a couple of months until heat-treated products were available.

Commission lawyer Marlys Edwardh prodded further. The message Schroeder had given at the time was that a change would have been difficult.

"It may have been understood that way," Schroeder replied. "It was not meant to be understood that way. I am aware the treaters knew we could provide cryoprecipitate." She said she had been told hemophiliacs did not want to switch back to cryo.

There were no requests, CHS lawyer Bonnie Tough remarked, because hemophiliacs had been told that an adequate supply was logistically impossible. The irony is that Schroeder was one of many doctors who believed cryo was a safer product.

The use of Canadian-source plasma concentrates was another option. The belief was it would be safer because it came from volunteer donors rather than commercial sources. This proved to be true. Nova Scotia, which used 100 per cent Canadian-source concentrates, ended up with the lowest HIV-infection rate for hemophiliacs among the provinces.

Some people in other provinces followed that pattern. Barry Isaac, a Calgary hemophiliac, decided as far back as 1981 that he would not use any American-source products. His concern at that time was actually hepatitis infection from paid-donor plasma, but his decision may have saved him from being infected with HIV. "I told our clinic that I just wouldn't take the stuff, and they said, 'Well, okay, but it's going to be inconvenient.' And I said, 'I don't care.' So whenever they were out of Canadian-source concentrates, I just went back to cryo."

Perrault's comments to the Commons sub-committee about the availability of cryoprecipitate shocked and angered Dr. Michelle Brill-Edwards, a professional regulator. "There were certain parts of the testimony where I had to stop reading and get up and walk around for a bit, because I realized that a thousand people are dying simply because these decisions were just shoved under the carpet!"

What of the role of the federal Bureau of Biologics, the regulator? Did they have any duty to suggest an alternative to a risky product?

Dr. Wark Boucher, the Bureau acting director in 1993 and chief of the blood division in the early 1980s, attempted to distance regulators from decisions on choice of product. "We regulate the safety. We're really not the treaters," he told the parliamentary subcommittee headed by Dr. Stan Wilbee. "The decision was that there should be non-heat-treated material available for those critical situations where you may have a serious bleeding episode," said Boucher. "Non-heat-treated material would be used if heat-treated wasn't available or if cryoprecipitate wouldn't suffice."

Dr. Rey Pagtakhan, a Liberal MP, said he found it "alarming" that use of unsafe products could still be permitted. Janice Hopkins, executive director in March 1993 of the federal Health Protection Branch, said the Bureau of Biologics had power to compel a manufacturer to take a product from the market. "The decision has to be carefully considered before removing the only [available] product from the market. So the decision is certainly tempered by whether there are other products available in sufficient quantity to replace the product in question."

Brill-Edwards expresses frustration at this regulatory approach. "The job of the Bureau, in the face of a health hazard, is to ascertain what alternative products could be available. We are the national agency. We are the watchdog. And if we're thinking of taking something off the market, it's part of our job to ascertain what alternative product is there to keep people alive. For me, it's a blasphemy for this agency to virtually lie to the professionals to say: 'Well, it's virtually all or nothing. Take it or leave it.' And then, of course, [the CHS medical and scientific advisory] committee begs and says: 'God, don't take it all away if we have nothing to replace it with.' So they were lying on two counts. They were lying when they said it was either all or none. And they were lying when they said there was no alternative available."

The testimony of Roger Perrault and others challenges the assertion by Bureau officials that in the critical period there was no alternative to non-heat-treated products. As they made clear, there was another product that could have been available in sufficient amounts until heat-treated concentrates became more widely available: cryoprecipitate.

There were other options to safeguard the system, too. These may not have been foolproof but might have increased safety. One option was to use a surrogate test for hepatitis B to screen out high-risk donors. Often, the same populations in which AIDS was showing up were also subject to hepatitis. If hepatitis-positive donations had been destroyed, much of the HIV-tainted blood would have been eliminated from the system along with them. A second option could have been to manufacture concentrates from smaller donor pools, rather than the giant pools of up to 25,000 sometimes used. For mild hemophiliacs with borderline coagulation defects, a compound known as desmopressin or DDAVP could have been used to unlock existing but non-active clotting capacity. In fact, Dr. Gail Rock, medical director of the Red Cross's Ottawa blood centre, had found that the use of this agent considerably increased the yields of clotting factor from plasma.

Another choice was reduced usage, yet this raised a dilemma. National medical advisors to the Canadian Hemophilia Society said concentrate should be used early to treat bleeds, thereby preventing an emerging hemorrhage from getting worse. If a bleed got out of hand, it would require much larger amounts of clotting factor. Prompt use of concentrate at the earliest possible moment might halt an episode in its tracks, but it meant treatment with whatever products were on hand.

Brill-Edwards, who was at Toronto's Hospital for Sick Children at the time and went on to work for the federal Health Protection Branch, disagrees with that advice. "It was appropriate when there was no risk of fatal contamination. But I think that [warning] signal could have been sent out in 1983, before we even discovered the virus. We knew this was a blood-borne disease. And it would have been a sensible precautionary measure to take, to say: 'Be careful. Raise your threshold of concern before you use this product.' "

Some hemophiliacs may have been warned off use of concentrates privately at the same time that doctors and the Red Cross were publicly urging them to carry on normal use. John Wilson, an Ottawa hemophiliac who at the time was making regular donations for research purposes, says he recalls being told by Perrault not to take concentrates unnecessarily. "We can't be sure of their safety," he quotes Perrault as saying. Wilson later became HIV-positive.

An innovative suggestion in 1984–85 that got the dust rising among doctors and Red Cross bureaucrats was a proposal that emerged from the Ontario wing of the Canadian Hemophilia Society, specifically Bill Mindell of Toronto. Mindell was then director of health information with the city and father of a young hemophiliac. He was also on the board of the provincial chapter. An intense, weedy man with a greying beard, Mindell has a master's degree in public health from the University of Michigan and had closely followed the spread of AIDS both in his work and out of personal interest.

Late in 1983 or in early 1984 Mindell had raised with Red Cross officials the possibility of using only female-donor blood as a source of cryoprecipitate. The idea was discouraged. Women were only 40 per cent of blood donors, he was told. Female donors were rejected more often than males because of low hemoglobin rates. He bought the argument "hook, line, and sinker" that a female-only system would not work, he says today.

A talk with a gay man at a meeting in the fall of 1984 revived the idea for him. "He was really concerned, and he said, 'What can we do about this hemophilia thing?' And I said, 'Well, it's easy. You just use women's blood.' And he said, 'Why don't you just have a lesbian blood drive?' " Mindell responded with all the reasons that had been quoted to him, but he couldn't shake the idea from his head.

The logic for the suggestion was simple. Mindell noted that in the latter half of 1984, there were only eleven documented cases of women with AIDS in Canada. Eight of them were Haitian immigrants, one was a Canadian-born woman who had lived twenty years in Haiti, and another had lived in Canada with several Haitian men. The only female AIDS victim without a Haitian connection was an American-born intravenous drug user. "Even if it wasn't absolutely safe, if you weren't Haitian and you were a woman in Canada, you were probably pretty safe, at least relatively safe compared to everyone else."

Mindell was pleased with himself. "It sounded to me the most brilliant idea I ever had. An elegant solution." Blood collection centres wouldn't have to ask embarrassing questions. There was enough female blood donated to supply the needs of hemophiliacs using cryo, so extra recruitment wouldn't be necessary. The other components, such as albumin and red blood cells, would still be available. It looked like a winner.

Mindell's "female donors only" idea was one of the few innovative proposals to surface at the time. The official parties — governments, the Red Cross, and the medical professions — had been curiously devoid of ideas. Mindell's proposal was also supported as theoretically sound by considerable numbers of doctors who regularly treated hemophiliacs.

Mindell developed the concept in November 1984 and enlisted the support of Dr. Abraham Shore, a doctor who worked at the Hospital for Sick Children and a hemophiliac, and Dr. Jerome Teitel, of the Hemophilia Comprehensive Care Clinic at St. Michael's Hospital in Toronto. Shore was enthusiastic and suggested the proposal be offered to the Red Cross. "They've been getting such bad press lately. We will just tell them they can have the idea."

Mindell approached Dr. Derek Naylor of the Red Cross. "It was offered as a strategy to the Canadian Red Cross Blood Transfusion Service for which they could take complete credit, including the original concept," Mindell wrote in July 1985. The proposal was also discussed with Roger Perrault. "Dr. Perrault agreed that it was sound epidemiologically but told me that he would have to wait and see what our MSAC would have to say about it." Mindell worked on the theme, writing and redrafting the proposal four times, incorporating many outside comments. It was sent with the Hemophilia Society's representatives to the consensus conference on December 10, 1984. This was the meeting that set out the timetable for distribution of the heat-treated products and turned over to the Society's MSAC the tough decisions of who would first get the new coagulants.

The paper was not distributed at the consensus conference, nor was the suggestion even raised. Later, Mindell was to write philosophically about the fact that the idea had not been discussed: "It was a crowded agenda for one day and had to deal with the important issue of heat-treated products."

That didn't mean he or his partners were about to quit. Less than two weeks after the conference, Mindell, Shore, and Teitel sent their proposal to the British medical journal *Lancet.* It appeared as a letter in the January 12, 1985, issue. The three men identified themselves by their occupations.

The letter said hemophiliacs were an HIV high-risk group that had no choice but to continue using the therapy that put them at risk. Hemophiliacs, and the doctors treating them, were confronted with a situation demanding that "all reasonable precautions" be taken in the processing of cryoprecipitate. They pointed out that in Canada there was no increase in the number of women who had developed AIDS in seven months. On the other hand, in the same period from May 17 to December 18, 1984, the number of males with AIDS had nearly doubled to 151. Furthermore, while 40 per cent of blood donations in Canada were made by women, less than half of those would be needed to make cryoprecipitate.

"We propose that processing all cryoprecipitates exclusively from female donors is a cost-effective strategy which will reduce the risk of AIDS to cryoprecipitate users," the letter said. Mindell, Shore, and Teitel said the proposal could be implemented immediately and would not require additional resources or personnel. "It would provide a window of relative safety from exposure to AIDS until more definitive alternatives are available."

The idea was attracting widespread interest. Dr. Irwin Walker, chairman of Hemophilia Ontario's medical and scientific advisory committee, wrote Mindell in December 1984 to say that he had contacted ten of the other twelve physicians on the committee. Nine supported the proposal, while the tenth expressed doubts.

Gordon Jessamine of the federal government's Laboratory Centre for Disease Control wrote Mindell the same month to say the idea was appropriate, timely, and well thought out. "It appears to be the most successful way of reducing the risk of infection — even maybe eliminating it entirely," Jessamine wrote. He did have one reservation: "We are just a little concerned that they [Canadian females] may not be as 'virginal' as your theoretical presentation suggests. You may be right, but it would be nice to be sure." Mindell also obtained support in a letter from Dr. Louis Aledort, an eminent American hematologist and hemophilia specialist.

Although the editors of *Lancet* thought the proposal of sufficient interest to publish it, back home in Canada the idea was treated with scorn by Red Cross authorities who apparently thought the lay population was getting uppity. Mindell's hitherto good relations with the Red Cross took a bad turn.

"All of a sudden there was cut-off," he says. "They weren't really very happy to see me when I walked around there after that. I got the cold shoulder. I spent the next few years really mad at them and feeling desperate and in despair. I had long gone past the point of realizing what a tragedy this whole thing was. I was quite hysterical. I wrote letters to everybody and you can see the anger in the letters, the frustration."

Mindell, as the father of a hemophiliac, and Shore, a hemophiliac himself, were accused of misrepresenting their interest by signing their professional affiliations to the letter rather than their personal connections. Derek Naylor openly criticized Mindell for using "unauthorized" statistics on the proportion of female donors. It actually was between 26 and 36 per cent, said Naylor. Mindell pointed out that didn't matter; all the proposal required was 20 per cent female donors.

Despite the attacks, the backers of the alternative cryoprecipitate proposal continued the battle. They also expanded their idea of safe cryoprecipitate sources. Some areas of the country — St. John's, Saskatoon, and Winnipeg, for instance — had not reported any AIDS cases, and it was believed these might be safer sources than the cities of Toronto, Montreal, and Vancouver. "Make the rest of the country bleed for a change," Mindell says today. "Just before the introduction of heat-treated products, I don't think I would have accepted anything less than female cryo from Northern Ontario."

Meanwhile, in early 1985 Shore presented the case to a meeting of blood fractionators, suppliers, and "users" (doctors and clinic representatives, not hemophiliacs), who requested more information.

In February, the Canadian Hemophilia Society's national blood resources committee endorsed the proposal. The suggestion then went before a meeting of Hemophilia Ontario's medical and scientific advisory committee, which included representatives of the Red Cross.

The Ontario MSAC meeting in late March 1985 was an unusual one. Families of hemophiliacs turned up. According to Bob O'Neill, who attended the session, the main item on the agenda was "safe cryo" as an immediate alternative. The Red Cross's Naylor, despite knowing what would be discussed, said he did not have necessary facts with him. Among the requested material was an estimate of possible increased costs arising from implementation of the proposal. Although this was supposedly one reason for the reluctance by the Red Cross to adopt the idea, no evidence of significant cost arising from the identification and separation was ever supplied over the eight months the issue was discussed. The Red Cross argument about higher costs and difficulties in physically separating male from female blood was never proven. It seems to have been a red herring.

The female-donor proposal found both supporters and detractors among the doctors at the Ontario MSAC meeting. Finally, a motion was approved asking the Red Cross's Naylor to supply information on the feasibility of the proposal. Naylor maintained his argument that it would not be possible to separate female from male blood donations without great cost. Mindell offered to provide seventeen Magic Markers, one for each regional centre, so that "F" could be marked on the bags. Naylor said separate refrigeration facilities would be needed. "Why would you need to do that?" asked Mindell. "None of it made sense."

Naylor's assertions were also challenged by O'Neill, who had worked in blood donor recruitment in Nova Scotia. "I said, sure it's feasible. Just put a sticker with an 'F' on the bags. It wouldn't cost anything." O'Neill says Naylor's face turned deep red.

The imagination of opponents to the safe-cryo proposal appeared to know no bounds. The Red Cross was joined by some federal authorities and doctors who doubted the idea would work and felt it would cause problems in the national blood system. Bob Gibson, a hemophiliac who later compiled a history of the affair for the Canadian Hemophilia Society, listed seven arguments against the proposal, including the supposed increase in cost and the feasibility of separating male from female donations. Some of these reasons were patently absurd, others contradictory.

Alistair Clayton of the Laboratory Centre for Disease Control voiced several. Male blood donors, he claimed, might stop giving blood because they would feel discriminated against. Furthermore, he wrote in a letter to Mindell, there was no scientific proof that people who were HIV-positive actually were infectious or carriers of the AIDS virus. Also, he argued, there was not enough knowledge yet about whether women with multiple sex partners would carry the virus. "I personally speculate that the next well-defined high-risk group is going to be female prostitutes," he said, with a degree of foresight.

Clayton carried his concerns a step further in a letter to Dr. Robert Card, the chairman of the national MSAC. There was also no scientific evidence that male donors presented a greater risk in HIV transmission, he wrote. Red Cross officials added their view that there had been no "documented" case of AIDS transmission through blood in Canada. This, Gibson commented, implied there was no urgency to the plan.

Two other criticisms related to the impact on the blood supply of separating female blood from that given by male donors. If plasma collected from women was removed from the pool and used for cryoprecipitate, that would mean the freeze-dried concentrates could be at greater risk because plasma from men — with an apparent infection rate ten times greater — would be a higher percentage of the pool. This argument contradicted those who suggested males were no more prone to contribute tainted blood than women. Ironically, in a roundabout way it was an argument in favour of using female blood. The epidemiological evidence was that only a tiny amount of blood could contaminate a large pool, so it was unlikely a decreased number of female donations in the plasma pool would make much difference.

The second argument was that if it was correct that female blood was less likely to be infected, then the entire supply should be collected from women only. And, if that was the case, questions would arise as to who would receive the blood in times of shortages. First, this was a hypothetical issue as there was no shortage. And second, when blood is received, no one asks its origins. If black Canadians happen to make more donations than whites, for example, does this mean supplies should be apportioned by race? Or should need prevail?

How did the supporters of these criticisms respond?

Gibson suggested that the continuing question of scientific proof of AIDS transmission through blood should have been irrelevant. "The AIDS situation, in 1984 and 1985 as now, was seen as urgent enough to warrant pragmatic approaches to its containment, even without conclusive clinical confirmation of specific phenomena." As experienced regulators agree, you act to eliminate the danger first, particularly when alternatives are available.

If the end users of these blood products got no satisfaction at the Ontario MSAC, they received an even cooler reception at the national MSAC meeting a month later. Mindell and other promoters of the safe-cryo idea were barred from the meeting, although officials from the Red Cross were there in force. Without the proponents inside the meeting, the proposal was never even discussed.

Mindell didn't give up, although by the beginning of May 1985 heat-treated concentrates were starting to be distributed. He was invited to appear on a panel during Toronto's AIDS Awareness Week to talk about AIDS and blood. Another panelist was to be John Derrick of the Red Cross, but Derrick never confirmed his attendance or returned calls to organizers. The panel, to be held June 10, was cancelled. The next day, the *Toronto Sun* asked Derrick why he had not agreed to participate. "He [Mindell] is beating a drum we're not dancing to," said Derrick.

Mindell acknowledges today that cryo was not without its problems. There are success stories where people switched and aren't infected, he says, but there is another side, too. "In my little cohort of friends, a lot of those had switched and have long been dead, whereas the ones who were infected through concentrates were up there testifying and they looked pretty good." Even though cryo was safer, for a severe hemophiliac to switch would mean using 1,000 to 1,500 bags of cryo a year with exposure to a lot of unprocessed protein, and a lot of potential reactions.

Mindell was bitter about the response to the proposal when he made a radical call for action in July 1985. "We have tried everything we can within the system to get action on safe cryo. We have waited, gotten encouraging words and uniform commitments, but no action," Mindell wrote in a confidential memo to the Hemophilia Ontario board. He felt the Red Cross blood transfusion service had labelled him an isolated crank, and said the lack of vigorous advocacy — and in some cases opposition — by doctors on the MSACs had hindered the proposal.

"I believe there are lives, and the quality of lives, at stake here. If the policies and recommendations I have been pushing are incorrect, we gain or lose nothing. If the present policies of the [Red Cross] are incorrect, we lose everything."

Mindell added several more suggestions to his proposal for collection of cryoprecipitate from women and safe regions. He called for directed donations from safe donors to hemophiliac patients and urged, impractically, the families of all hemophiliacs to move to AIDS-free areas of the country. He called for the adoption of stricter donor screening and donor blood designations already adopted in the U.S. Mindell also requested donations to help the Canadian Hemophilia Society set up an alternative blood collection system to the Red Cross.

He ended with a declaration: "We hold the Canadian Red Cross blood transfusion service responsible for every cryo user who goes [HIV] positive after the initial round of tests now being conducted."

Even today, when Mindell's view of the Red Cross has moderated, he remembers how exasperated he felt.

"I can't tell you how frustrating it was. I felt like I was pouring sand into the ocean."

The Red Cross seems to have been distressingly dismissive of ideas that emerged from the consumer group they were supposed to be working for. But that was only a continuation of their approach throughout the affair.

Red Cross officials had questioned the right of consumers of blood products to have their say on the best ways to avoid blood contamination. The suggestions were labelled emotional and biased. Mindell and Shore had been attacked because they had a personal involvement and weren't perceived, therefore, as rational and scientific. Yet the editors of *Lancet* had seen merit in the safe-cryo idea and had given it full exposure.

"They didn't feel they should be responding to scientific proposals from the lay population," says Bob O'Neill. "John Derrick said to me, 'These proposals should be coming from the medical and scientific advisory committee, not you.'" The trouble is, the MSAC seemed little inclined to push the idea.

O'Neill says Red Cross officials held the view that the families who pushed for the safe-cryo proposal were over-reacting. They said society members were "biased because of their personal involvement and weren't seeing things rationally." But O'Neill points out that "the first person to recognize there is a problem is the person who is directly affected."

Many hemophiliacs, and no doubt those who suffer from other chronic afflictions, would recognize the kind of paternalistic brush-off given the safe-cryo proposal. It's the kind of nonsense they are used to hearing all their lives. If doctors, regulators, and other officials would listen more often, then the quality of the lives of the chronically ill — and those who treat them — would be far better.

Chapter 7

THE POLITICS OF A WASTED RESOURCE

*"How many parents are out there wondering what is wrong
with their child, running off to a doctor who, in turn,
is not able to pinpoint the illness? Why is this product available
if it is causing so many ill side effects?"*

MOTHER OF A SIX-YEAR-OLD HEMOPHILIAC, 1988

One of the most political and self-serving decisions in the tainted
blood scandal was the insistence by the Ontario government that
Connaught Laboratories of Toronto be given a monopoly in the
province over production of Factor VIII concentrate from volunteer-
donated plasma. The aims were to make Canada self-sufficient and
to create jobs. But it ended up achieving neither of those goals at the
expense of consumer safety. It was political favouritism gone haywire.

Connaught, theoretically, looked like the right company for the
job of making blood products. The Canadian-owned company's roots
dated back to 1917, when it was established as a medical research laboratory of the University of Toronto to produce vaccines and serums.
In that capacity, its reputation grew. It produced insulin for diabetics
after Frederick Banting and Charles Best discovered the vital medication that saved so many lives. It became the largest Canadian manufacturer of biological products. Profits were reinvested in research. In
1954, after heroic work during the war years, it established a plant to
fractionate blood, splitting plasma into needed components.

Through its involvement in the blood system, Connaught had
close ties with the Red Cross, including a contract for plasma fractionation. Some connections were not entirely aboveboard. There

was reportedly a "gentlemen's agreement" between the two agencies in the 1960s and early 1970s which was never made public. Over thirteen years, for instance, Connaught sold blood products worth nearly $7 million and the Red Cross got a 10 per-cent cut of the action. Some of these components were exported, and in the mid-70s journalists stumbled across evidence that one product used in the treatment of burns, serum albumin, was being sold abroad just as a shortage was developing in Canada. The sale of a scarce product was denied as a "gross inaccuracy," but soon after the $500,000 transaction there was suddenly a lack of serum albumin in Canada. The Red Cross in November 1974 was able to supply only about one-third of the orders. "It was a freak thing," a Connaught apologist said. Extraordinary or not, Ottawa stepped in and banned the export of albumin.

Relations between the two entities had already started to crumble when the serum albumin issue surfaced. In 1972, the University of Toronto had sold Connaught to the Canada Development Corporation, a company in which the federal government was the largest single shareholder.

"Prior to 1972, the Canadian Red Cross and Connaught Laboratories appeared to have had a good cooperative relationship," said a 1980 report on plasma fractionation prepared under the direction of Chapin Key, British Columbia's deputy health minister. The Red Cross would collect whole blood, do primary processing, transfer raw materials to Connaught for secondary processing, and distribute the products to Canadian hospitals. The provinces, on a formula proportionate to population, would pay the Red Cross, and it would in turn reach contracted deals with processors. The report went on to say that "After 1972, when Connaught Laboratories came under the aegis of the Canada Development Corporation, cooperation tended to deteriorate." Federal-provincial committees were established, at least in part to resolve growing disputes over blood collection, processing, and distribution.

Meanwhile, many observers of the blood industry had misgivings about Connaught's capability to produce suitable blood products. Its facilities were aging and there were problems of contamination of some products. Federal inspections found Connaught had failed to meet quality control and other standards. In 1975, a series of articles in the *Globe and Mail* cited violations of federal rules, contamination, and danger of infection. A Connaught executive conceded government standards were not being met. As much as half of the whole blood Connaught received was not completely fractionated because it was contaminated in processing.

Dr. Cecil Harris of Montreal, who had worked for many years as a professional and volunteer in blood banking and hemophilia, was one of the critics. The honorary life member of the Canadian Hemophilia Society wrote the *Medical Post* in 1977 to say Connaught should be phased out of plasma fractionation.

Even senior Connaught executives were concerned. Dr. Andrew Moriarty, a vice-president of the parent company, said the plant needed to be reconstructed. Expansion of the existing fractionation plant was a waste of time. Moriarty was fired for his impudence.

Connaught's production was also expensive. Dr. Roger Perrault of the Red Cross told *Maclean's* magazine in 1976 that the profit motive was very much in evidence at Connaught. The federal government, trying to attract private investors, wanted the crown corporation to pay more attention to the bottom line. But the Red Cross had found that 40 per cent of the fresh-frozen plasma it sent to Connaught for fractionation had to be destroyed owing to contamination. That year, Red Cross officials advanced the notion that they should have their own $10-million fractionating plant built, and ties with Connaught should be cut. This, they said, would be the best way for Canada to achieve self-sufficiency in blood and its derivatives.

There was some support given to the Red Cross idea by the Canadian Hemophilia Society. Hemophiliacs wanted a fractionation plant in Canada in the 1970s, too, but had reservations about Connaught. A more sophisticated plant would be needed to produce blood factor concentrates. Another compelling reason for opposition to Connaught among hemophiliacs was that in pursuit of the bottom line,

Connaught had suggested using paid donor plasma. Donors motivated by financial reward, rather than the spirit of giving, could pose a risk to the system. (Pointed evidence they were right, too late for many AIDS victims, came a decade later when it was noted that those countries and provinces that used larger amounts of imported commercially produced American factor, had higher rates of HIV infection.)

The qualified view of the Canadian Hemophilia Society was that national self-sufficiency was desirable — but not at the expense of reliable and safe production. Its leaders feared supplies of quality Factor VIII concentrate would be jeopardized if politicians chose an inefficient but homebred fractionating company over an efficient U.S. producer making products from Canadian blood shipped south by the Red Cross.

Unfortunately, the way the desirable concept of self-sufficiency was implemented backfired on the safety of Canada's blood supply.

The strongest political proponent of self-sufficiency was the Conservative government of Ontario. Connaught's plant was located in Metro Toronto's Willowdale district, next door to the riding of Dennis Timbrell, then Ontario's health minister.

Timbrell was a politician with clout. And he made clear his position in an October 1979 letter to Elie Martel, an opposition member of the provincial legislature. A concerned member of the Hemophilia Society had written Martel asking for help. Timbrell dismissed the concerns as "misinformation."

"My ministry position is that we have an efficient and sufficient fractionation facility here in Canada available to supply virtually all our needs," Timbrell wrote. He added that Connaught was operating at half capacity because of lack of supply from the Red Cross; he wanted a majority, if not all, of donated blood sent there for processing.

"The question of building a new fractionation facility at a cost of many millions is quite unnecessary," Timbrell said. "This will ensure the best possible supply at the least possible cost in Canada, the essential answers to the questions of every hemophiliac."

Connaught Labs and Timbrell launched an attack on the Red Cross for signing, in the summer of 1980, a thirty-two-month contract with Cutter Laboratories, a California-based firm, which would produce concentrated clotting factor from Canadian plasma. Connaught caught Timbrell's ear when it complained. "At this point Connaught Laboratories, supported by the Ministry of Health in Ontario, expressed concern publicly that Canadian blood was being shipped outside of Canada for fractionation, to the detriment of the only plant and personnel in Canada which had the technical capability of achieving self-sufficiency in production for the Canadian public," the 1980 Key report said. It added drolly that the rival companies, Connaught and Cutter, were both in the business of making money.

Timbrell sketched a scary scenario in which the Americans, in times of shortage, might seize Canadian-origin plasma for their own use. The Red Cross responded that in the event of emergency what might happen is that Canadian plasma would have a lower priority for processing than the American equivalent. If that "remote possibility" did occur, the Canadian Red Cross would revert to production of cryoprecipitate, the less pure but "adequate" product that many hemophiliacs had used for years. The country could be self-sufficient in cryoprecipitate.

The Red Cross also defended the Cutter deal by pointing out that until 1979 — when Connaught got its licence to produce concentrates — there was no facility in Canada. Canadian plasma had been sent south by the Red Cross for processing beginning in 1978. And the Red Cross signed with Cutter with the backing of a federal-provincial government committee.

The Cutter contract provided for the production of clotting factor from 245,000 litres of Canadian fresh-frozen plasma, shipped south and returned, for $9.1 million. Connaught, the Red Cross pointed out, had asked for $13.5 million for the same output. Furthermore, Timbrell's favourite had demanded an annual increment equal to 10 per cent above the inflation rate and an incentive clause for yields above a guaranteed minimum. These were pretty extravagant demands from a company that had yet to prove it could produce any Factor VIII.

Connaught knew it had the political edge, and it pushed its case. Timbrell made no pretence of neutrality. It would be worth paying the extra $5 million to process in Canada, he said.

Hemophiliacs, however, were troubled. "We are appalled by Connaught's stated intention to purchase blood with all the consequences of higher costs and products contaminated by hepatitis and other diseases," the CHS Ontario president, Frank Terpstra, wrote to Timbrell in September 1980. "We cannot help but see serious implications for future supply in commercialization of blood products." He asked Timbrell to reconsider his position for the sake of hemophiliacs and consumers of other blood products.

Chapin Key and his committee surveyed all of this argument and counter-argument. "There appear to be considerable emotional issues being debated publicly in the area of self-sufficiency and gratuity of profit," the Key report said. "The presence of personality conflicts is possibly a basis for this poor communication and philosophical difference."

Connaught won out. The provinces spurned the Red Cross proposal to build its own plant. The Canadian Blood Committee ordered the Red Cross to break its contract with Cutter. All of Ontario's plasma and some from other provinces was sent to Connaught. Timbrell's pet was given a monopoly for production of Factor VIII in Ontario and gained access as well to government funds for research in the area of blood products. The Institut Armand Frappier in Quebec was approved for production of concentrates from plasma on a non-profit basis. The Rh Institute in Winnipeg was designated for specialized fractionation. The Red Cross retained its distributive role and could renegotiate contracts with Cutter until such time as the country was self-sufficient. Meanwhile, some of the plasma the Red Cross collected from other provinces was sent to Cutter for processing.

It didn't take long for problems to show up. Connaught's plant was the oldest in North America. The facility was described by visitors as aging, smelly, decrepit, and dirty. The Factor VIII produced was of poor quality and yields were about a third lower than that produced by its American counterparts. Some people found dark foreign objects, probably rubber particles, floating in the reconstituted product that they were expected to inject into their veins. Among the complaints from users were hives, chills, and light-headedness. One London, Ontario, hemophiliac reported "consistent mild reactions" with use of Connaught clotting factor. "With each treatment I have considerable pain around the puncture site with redness that appears approximately fifteen to twenty minutes after the needle has been removed," he said. In some cases, he felt sharp pain. "It has inhibited my willingness to receive prompt infusions." He added, "I look forward to receiving the results and learning what the small black particle was."

Bill Mindell, then head of CHS Ontario's factor products committee, says the Red Cross hated their forced relationship with Connaught. "They hated the fact that they were sending all this great plasma over there and Connaught was blowing it. The Red Cross had to continue to deliver and pay for product that they never received. Eventually a settlement was reached where Connaught paid them back for the product that was never delivered. But the plasma was lost."

In October 1981, Red Cross officials met with Connaught counterparts to discuss the user complaints. John Derrick of the Red Cross noted that rubber particles had appeared in some other Connaught products. "By contrast, no such contamination appears to occur with Hyland or Cutter products," Derrick said, according to a meeting summary. Connaught agreed to solve the problem of rubber particles getting into the vials but defended itself by blaming the users. They were probably not reconstituting the product properly, it said; Connaught would reinforce the necessity of following instructions.

That meeting failed to resolve the continuing difficulties with the Connaught product. There were two recalls for hepatitis contamination in the late summer of 1983. Two donors, who had made four donations between them, had "forgotten" to tell the blood collection stations in the United States where Connaught obtained some of its plasma that they had hepatitis infections five years before. The recalls, said Jo-Anne Harper, program director for Hemophilia Ontario, had led the Red Cross to cancel a supplementary contract with Connaught and turn to the U.S. firms Cutter and Hyland for supply.

"The last three consecutive batches of Canadian-source plasma Factor VIII concentrate that Connaught has fractionated have not met minimum standards for solubility, and as a result, have had to be re-processed," she wrote in a November 1983 letter. "Not only has the yield been dramatically reduced, but there has been and will be for some time virtually no Canadian-source Factor VIII concentrate available in southern Ontario."

The problem of solubility of the powder concentrate in saline solution continued to plague Connaught. It sometimes took an hour to dissolve the concentrate in saline before injections. Some consumers reported they were afraid to use the company's product. Hemophiliacs suffered because they faced unnecessary damage and pain while they waited for the product to dissolve properly before injection.

Perhaps the worst impact was the continuing inability of Connaught to produce adequate amounts of good-quality Factor VIII in an efficient manner. This meant that to have sufficient supply the company had to fall back on American plasma from the blood of paid donors. One of Connaught's plasma suppliers in the United States was rumoured to have collected blood from the prison system, a notorious haven for diseases like hepatitis. And that situation was exactly what the supporters of Canadian self-sufficiency had hoped to avoid.

Dr. Derek Naylor of the Red Cross, in a memo to medical directors of hemophilia clinics in August 1983, spoke of continuing technical problems in the production of Factor VIII concentrate by Connaught.

Still, government money kept rolling into Connaught's coffers. The company received nearly $9 million from the federal government in 1982 for research into the production of Factor VIII through gene splicing. It received another $2 million the same year from Ontario to replace the outdated Willowdale plant.

By October 1983, Ontario had a new health minister, Keith Norton. At a meeting between Norton, Hemophilia Society representatives, and the AIDS Committee of Toronto, it was reported that Connaught had, in one year, lost a five-month supply of donated Canadian plasma, sufficient to supply all of Ontario's Factor VIII needs. Over three years, the losses equalled one full year's supply, or the equivalent of 215,000 blood donations. The total value of those donations, Mindell estimated, was $13 million. Since Factor VIII was about 15 per cent of the blood products recovered from a donation, the losses in concentrate alone amounted to about $2 million. And what was produced was of such poor quality that much of it had to be reprocessed.

A year later, nothing had improved. When Naylor told Hemophilia Society representatives that the usual two-month reserve of Factor VIII had dropped to two weeks, he mentioned the Connaught debacle as a primary cause.

Connaught, he told Mindell, had run into major production difficulties. They had ceased fractionation of plasma in April 1984 and had stockpiled cryoprecipitate for six months. While stored, the frozen cryoprecipitate had lost its potency as well.

Earlier, Naylor told his Red Cross colleague Dr. Roger Perrault that his experts had been working with Connaught technical representatives since 1981 to overcome problems of minimum contract yields, varying product quality, and infrequent deliveries. "No measurable progress has been made in resolving them," Naylor's memo said, "and this perhaps is attributable to the limited resources available to Connaught's plasma products division."

Mindell, getting a rundown on Connaught's problems, called for the termination of the Red Cross–Connaught contract and the immediate diversion of all Canadian plasma and cryoprecipitate to an approved American fractionator. There were 12,000 litres of unprocessed cryoprecipitate. "They could give it to the Rh Institute in Winnipeg to practise with, but it won't be used therapeutically," said an angry Mindell.

He had also received reports from consumers of shortcomings in Connaught's products. In October 1984, Ottawa hemophiliacs were still reporting dizziness, shortness of breath, flushing, and pounding in the veins. "Will use Connaught if nothing else available," one user reported. "Will not use Connaught under any circumstance," said another. "Conversations with Red Cross lead me to understand that many (if not most) area hemophiliacs experience reactions to Connaught Factors VIII and IX," reported Dan Huneault, who used the product himself. "However, most hemophiliacs tend to take the reactions as normal if minor and do not report them."

In November 1984, Mindell wrote that Connaught had much difficulty coming up with a product that met "minimal acceptable standards." Moreover, there was no evidence it was improving its capacity at a time when there was increasing hope for an artificial blood-clotting factor.

"If I was at Connaught now, I would consider it foolish to invest in current, near-obsolete technology with these changes on the horizon.

"Connaught has consistently demonstrated not only a lack of expertise in this field and the inability to produce an acceptable product for therapeutic use, but a total lack of corporate commitment to doing anything about it over the last four to five years. And that's in spite of the political backing and mandate they received!

"We're not just talking about another oil company here!" Mindell concluded, referring to the procession of oil companies taken over by governments during that period.

Mindell's remark about investing in obsolete technology was soon answered. After the federal Bureau of Biologics directed in November 1984 that all concentrates should be heat-treated, Connaught was told that no more fresh-frozen plasma from the Red Cross would be sent to the company for processing.

But that didn't slow down Connaught's executives. Bill Cochrane, the corporate chairman, appeared before the Canadian Blood Committee executive in January 1985 to complain that the decision would have a devastating impact on his company. The Bureau's decision was "premature," Cochrane said. Waving the flag of national self-sufficiency, Cochrane and a colleague then made a pitch for a "temporary relief package" from governments to offset Connaught's losses. The company's constant efforts to extract money from politicians seemed better developed than its ability to extract quality blood products.

When a new Liberal government took office in Ontario in mid-1985, Bob Pedersen, then president of the provincial Hemophilia Society, wrote the new health minister, Murray Elston, to put his concerns on the record. Self-sufficiency in Canadian plasma collection was a far more urgent priority to hemophiliacs than where the blood was fractionated, Pedersen argued. Noting Connaught's serious difficulties, he pointed out that the company's failings had compelled use of riskier American products.

"Our Society has grave reservations about Connaught's ability to manage the production of a consistently high-quality product, and we strongly oppose a renewal of their fractionation contract until such time as they can demonstrate that they can do so competitively," Pedersen wrote. "Their demonstrated inefficiency . . . has been costly to Ontario hemophiliacs by increasing the reliance on hastily acquired, imported blood products, with the increased risk of exposure to deadly viruses." Pedersen added that past contract decisions seemed to have been based on economic criteria rather than health needs.

Elston's response, a month later, offered consultation, but he managed to avoid mentioning the Connaught situation even once. At the time, Connaught's plant had become so decrepit that the Bureau of Biologics threatened to revoke the company's licence.

Connaught's failure to produce came at the worst possible time for Canada's, and especially Ontario's, hemophiliacs. At a critical period, when HIV contamination was spreading in the blood supply, and before heat treatment, many of these people were given no choice but to use paid-donor U.S. products. In Ottawa, Toronto, and

Hamilton, only about 35 per cent of the concentrates used in 1983 came from Canadian volunteers. (Montreal was even lower at 29 per cent, but this was more because of heavy prophylaxis use than because of reliance on Connaught.) In other cities, the use of volunteer plasma from Canadian donors was considerably higher — a full 100 per cent in Halifax, 89 per cent in Calgary, and 77 per cent in Winnipeg.

Self-sufficiency continued to be a bugbear. Dr. Robert Card, chairman of the Canadian Hemophilia Society's Medical and Scientific Advisory Committee in March 1985, said Canadian fractionation should continue to be a desirable goal, if not possible at that time. "When new processes such as heat treating are introduced, we have virtually no clout with non-Canadian fractionators to ensure that Canadian hemophiliacs will be in the first groups to receive such advances."

The Canadian-owned fractionator also does not seem to have been terribly fussy about the plasma it would process. Dr. Noel Buskard, former medical director in British Columbia for the Red Cross, told the Krever blood commission that in the fall of 1985, untested plasma recalled from B.C. hospitals was shipped off to Connaught at the instruction of the Red Cross national office.

Normally, B.C. plasma was sent to the American firm Cutter, where it was processed into various blood products. But Cutter did not want anything to do with unscreened plasma coming from north of the border. Cutter had stringent requirements in the United States about the plasma they would fractionate, Buskard told Krever in April 1994. They were quite diligent and would not take the risky Canadian material. "I believe this would not pass muster for [Cutter]," Buskard added.

It seems to have been quite all right for blood users in Ontario.

Connaught, jumping back into the game after the advent of heat-treated concentrates, tried to come up with its own version. An announcement was made in June 1986, but a year later, hemophiliacs were still waiting. When Connaught's heat-processed concentrates did arrive, the same old complaints surfaced—nausea, faintness, flushing, and pain at the infusion site, and poor solubility.

One mother of a six-year-old boy wrote the Red Cross in January 1988 to complain that Connaught products were still causing problems. "I am upset because my son experienced extreme tiredness and a general feeling of malaise. He lost his appetite and complained of headaches. I am disappointed because the Canadian Red Cross Society is giving our hemophiliacs blood products that are causing many problems." She also related that she had difficulty dissolving the powder.

"How many parents are out there wondering what is wrong with their child, running off to a doctor who, in turn, is not able to pinpoint the illness?" she asked. "How do they find out the culprit is poor quality blood product? Why is this product available if it is causing so many ill side effects? What is the Red Cross going to do about it?"

Santo Caira, Hemophilia Ontario's AIDS coordinator for the Toronto region, was more blunt in an early 1988 letter. He had received complaints about Connaught's dry-heated concentrates, which were still in use. "The product is garbage. I've used it myself, and it's crap!" Caira exclaimed. "We have to act on this issue immediately. These bastards can't be allowed to walk away unscathed."

The idealized notion of Canadian self-sufficiency in blood products suffered a damaging blow from which it has not yet recovered. Nor did the other two proposed Canadian producers, the Rh Institute in Winnipeg and the Institut Armand Frappier in Quebec, do anything to cushion this dismal record—neither of them ever came up with any significant, marketable clotting concentrate.

The Red Cross placed its eggs chiefly in the Cutter basket. Its poor relations over many years with Connaught did not improve noticeably. Some of the same personalities were in control of the blood program who had been around since the Red Cross was denied its fractionation plant by the provincial governments. The bitter roots of that hostility seem to stick in the craw of Red Cross authorities even today. The provinces, with the exception of Nova Scotia, where the latest plan is to locate a $150-million plant, resisted construction of the proposed fractionator until a blue-ribbon committee studying the issue urged a go-ahead. The Canadian Blood Agency, the creature of the provinces that pays for approved blood products, is engaged in a continuing power struggle with the Red Cross. Miles Canada, with corporate ties to Cutter, is the Red Cross partner in the proposed Nova Scotia facility, which would be operated by a newly established corporation.

The experience of the past led the CBA to the view that self-sufficiency of Canadian blood products has nothing to do with where Canadian-source plasma is processed. The agency's executive director, William Dobson, told the Krever blood inquiry in February 1994 that the attempt by the provinces to divide Canada's production into three plants in the 1980s "destroyed any economies of scale."

Hemophilia Society officials had long abandoned the notion that this country needed to be self-sufficient in blood products fractionated in Canada. Society president Bob Pedersen told a meeting of blood experts early in 1988 that as technology improved, consumers wanted the best available concentrates immediately. "We do not care whether these products are made in Austria, New York, North Carolina, or Willowdale," Pedersen said. "But we're tired of having to infuse our children with a second-rate product just because it was made in Willowdale!"

Also significant in the self-sufficiency debacle was the loss of money the provincial governments suffered. The ill-fated Rh Institute experiment in Winnipeg cost the provinces $25 to $30 million, and only small amounts of blood products were ever distributed. The lesson provincial ministers derived from the failure, Dobson told the inquiry, was that if a plant was to be built, it should not be done by government.

That's one reason the CBA issued a direction in 1993 to the Red Cross to drop the idea of building a Canadian fractionation plant. While the deal would not involve taxpayers' funds up front, the proponents wanted commitments from the agency and the provinces that they would buy the products.

Because the Red Cross had no independent source of money for such a project, Dobson said the agency feared the provincial governments would be on the hook if something went wrong. He bluntly informed the Red Cross that the CBA would do everything in its power to block the project. The Red Cross has defiantly proceeded with plans for a plant to produce Factor VIII, albumin, immunoglobulin, and other products, and the cost may well surpass the estimate of $150 million. Dr. Maung Aye, Red Cross national director of blood services, says Miles Canada will "take off our hands" any product surplus. If there is no market in Canada, the blood derivatives will be sold to other countries, possibly to the Third World, which is desperately short of these products.

By 1987, troubled Connaught finally wanted out and quietly faded away from the clotting-factor business. "Subsequently, the Red Cross and Connaught reached an understanding that Connaught would be released from its contractual obligations to produce Factor VIII and Factor IX concentrates," wrote Bob Gibson, a hemophiliac who compiled a summary of the events of those tragic years.

Sanda Rodgers of the University of Ottawa's law faculty has investigated another factor in the demise of Connaught. After the AIDS scare had developed, Connaught refused to continue plasma fractionation unless the Red Cross and the provincial governments would cover any potential liability. "Finally, in June 1987, Connaught Laboratories informed the Canadian Blood Committee of its decision not to invest in a new fractionation facility," Rodgers wrote in a 1989 article. "The decision was based on the failure of the interested parties to provide Connaught with protection against liability for blood products and the fast-changing biotechnology that was likely to seriously affect blood products and make investment decisions exceedingly difficult." Connaught phased out, and new deals were arranged with American suppliers at a "substantial" saving to taxpayers.

It was good riddance. But the once-proud company had left a deplorable imprint on the lives of many Canadian hemophiliacs.

In an odd twist of fate, Connaught's ardent advocate Dennis Timbrell — reincarnated as head of the Ontario Hospital Association — wound up in 1994 advising patients who had blood transfusions between 1978 and 1985 to have themselves tested for HIV.

JOHN PLATER

John Plater, a tall, red-haired man in his mid-twenties, is studying law today. He remembers the snowy January morning in 1986 when his mother got the bad news at their home in Collingwood, Ontario.

"It was really stormy in the morning and the buses that took us to school weren't running. Halfway through the morning the phone rang and my mother called for me to come upstairs. She was upset and crying; it was the hemophilia clinic nurse at Sick Kids phoning to tell us."

Plater says when he went for his first clinic visit after the call, he was told that it was uncertain what a positive test meant. "Don't worry about it yet," they said. "We're pretty convinced that people are living longer with this. If you live five years, everything will be fine and it might not affect you."

Plater had been riding high then. He was student council president at his high school, he had his first serious girlfriend, and something inside him said he was going to miss this virus that people were talking about.

"So when my mother said the test was positive, it's not that the whole world came crashing down on me. I started thinking, I'll just play this as it goes. I've always had a deep faith, and what that's meant for me is that I don't get too worried about the future."

When high school ended, he went travelling in Europe with some friends. Another young hemophiliac who lived near Plater had developed full-blown AIDS. "It was weird, because he was a kid I'd known all my life. He was a bit younger than me, and our mothers were fairly close. It wasn't like he was a buddy of mine, but the whole trip it was in the back of my mind—how he was doing. "I'd always say a prayer when I went to see a cathedral. I'd just stop, and it was there."

JOHN WILSON

John Wilson, a hemophiliac from Osgoode, Ontario, near Ottawa, was told in early 1986 that he had tested positive for HIV antibodies. But he misinterpreted what that meant. He understood that he had been exposed to the virus, but thought the presence of antibodies meant his body had fought off the infection and he was, in effect, vaccinated and not capable of passing it on to others.

With what is known today, Wilson's belief may seem ingenuous. But at the time there was still much debate over what a positive antibody result meant. Michael O'Shaughnessy, who was director of the National Reference Laboratory for AIDS, told the Commons subcommittee on health issues that HIV represented a new class of human pathogens.

In diseases like measles and influenza, an antibody means you have been infected in the past or have been vaccinated. "For those who develop the antibody as a result of a natural infection, the virus usually disappears after the initial bout of the disease," O'Shaughnessy told the committee in March 1993. "So when you get sick with influenza, you make the antibody, and the virus disappears. You do not carry influenza. You carry the antibody, but that's not infectious."

With a so-called retrovirus like HIV, those with the antibody are not only infected, they are capable of passing the agent along. "We didn't have this information in 1984 and 1985," said O'Shaughnessy. "The other answers came three years later."

So, Wilson was not alone in his assumption that danger had passed him by. Many others trying to come to grips with the infection thought that way.

"It never sunk in any further than that," says Wilson, who lives on a small farm with his wife, Gudrun, and three sons. "I couldn't envision how a virus could go through the blood-fractionation process and still retain a virus's characteristics."

Wilson said it was another year before he had "proof positive" he was infectious. He had been regularly donating blood for some projects in which researchers were trying to grow infected cells in culture. He was invited by the hemophilia nurse at the Ottawa General Hospital to meet the doctor who was doing the work.

"She was trying to get me to come to grips with it. She realized this guy is not going to believe he is infected until he sees what the virus is doing to his cells. In those days, they didn't have psychologists to help you out, and the normal state of affairs for anyone who has a fatal illness is denial."

The doctor explained that he had petri dishes arranged on the near side of the table with infected cells, and on the other side with normal cells.

"I walked over to the other side of the table and I said, 'Where's my petri dish?' and he said, 'Sorry, John. You're on this side.'

"I had to have that physical proof and here it was—'J.W.' marked on the dish, and the doctor saying, 'These are your cells in culture, and you can see they are infected because of the abnormal clumping of the T-4 cells.' I talked to him for ten minutes or so, and then I walked out. A day or so later I said to myself, Shit, I guess I do have that virus in me."

Chapter 8

TOO LITTLE, TOO LATE

"There are two ways to scare a hemophiliac. One is to say the blood's bad and the other is to say there's no blood."

BILL MINDELL, FORMER CHAIR OF HEMOPHILIA ONTARIO'S
FACTOR PRODUCTS COMMITTEE, MAY 1994

The same month in mid-1984 that Dr. John Derrick of the Red Cross was playing down the risk of AIDS transmission through the blood supply in an article in the *Canadian Medical Association Journal*, tests done on blood from Canadian hemophiliacs had produced some startling results.

Dr. Michael O'Shaughnessy, then director of the federal Laboratory Centre for Disease Control, had been invited to train with Dr. Robert Gallo at the National Institutes of Health in the United States. In April, Gallo had discovered his HTLV-III virus, later found to be the same as the LAV virus previously discovered in France. O'Shaughnessy took with him large numbers of blood samples collected from gay men in Montreal and Toronto and a group of three to four hundred samples taken from hemophiliacs across the country. The testing was supervised by Chris Tsoukas of McGill University.

"Our initial findings in July and August 1984 were that many individuals with hemophilia were infected with HIV," O'Shaughnessy told the Commons sub-committee on health issues in March 1993. "In fact, more than half the samples I brought with me were positive." Later, he verified those findings at his Ottawa lab using the U.S.

techniques. The Ottawa lab was, at the time, the only testing site for the HIV antibody in Canada.

Hemophiliacs and blood transfusion patients still formed a very small proportion of those with AIDS. In November 1985, it was reported there were 231 adults with AIDS in Canada. The vast majority, 174, were gay men, followed by Haitians at 33 (plus 19 who did not fall into any high-risk category). There were three hemophiliacs and two recipients of transfused blood. There were also 17 children with AIDS—one was a blood recipient, the others had parents in "high-risk groups."

The researchers found that not all of the HIV-positive people tested were showing signs of AIDS. Instead of assuming—as others had—that this apparent good health meant that HIV-positivity was not a fatal condition, O'Shaughnessy judged that it would take some time for the immune disease to show up. "We found out then that you need not be sick if you were infected with this virus. So this was a very early clue that there was a long latency period. You could carry the antibody and appear healthy."

It took nearly a year after O'Shaughnessy's discovery for heat-treated blood products to be fully distributed to hemophiliacs. Once they were, there was a general recall of all non-heat-treated products from hospitals after July 1, 1985. The Red Cross also instructed the hospitals to ask hemophiliacs to return any non-heated products.

Most adult hemophiliacs and many older children had a stock of blood products at home, which they would use when a bleeding episode occurred. The patients were trained to mix up the concentrates or cryoprecipitate and inject themselves in a vein, usually in the elbow or the hand. In the case of younger children, their parents would do it for them, first learning how to find a vein by trying it on themselves. Often, parents were more adept at finding the elusive veins in a child's arm than doctors or nurses. They cared more, too, if there were problems, and they were more inclined to avoid inflicting needless pain on their child. Home care was a wonderful advancement.

For the hemophiliac, it meant no more sitting in growing pain during two-hour waits in hospital emergency rooms while inexperienced interns decided this test or that was required before blood products could be infused. Moreover, busy doctors and nurses could have more time to spend with other patients.

The blood products were obtained from hospital clinics or blood banks along with record sheets for home-care clients to log the details of each bleed, the lot numbers of manufactured products used, days lost at school or work, and other information. To get the products, all a hemophiliac had to do was to call the local clinic and request what he needed.

There were three levels of returns of blood products, each with different degrees of urgency. A "withdrawal" was a voluntary measure usually ordered by a manufacturer. A "replacement" occurred when the Red Cross took back questionable lots and substituted other material.

Sometimes, if a problem was identified in some distributed blood products, a "recall" would be necessary. Although the word is used loosely to refer to any return of products, a recall has specific meaning in that manufacturers might be legally liable. The recall could be ordered by either the Red Cross or the producer.

In some parts of Canada, little apparent distinction was made between the varying levels of urgency. Dr. Richard Huntsman, the medical director of the Newfoundland Red Cross transfusion service, told the Krever inquiry that all were treated as urgent and in the same manner: "effectively reaching for the phone."

Communication was critical. If word didn't get out quickly enough, a recall could fail, putting users' health at risk. To be effective, it should provoke an immediate response. Because blood products are often quickly used by patients, the vast majority of concentrates may be used before a notice is sent out. Authorities seem reluctant at times to use the appropriate terminology. At one point in 1987, when it was urgent to get dangerous products off hospital shelves, the Red Cross used the word "replacement," and some stock was evidently not returned for three to four weeks.

An example of a recall failure happened in September 1983, when Factor VIII concentrate produced by Connaught and contaminated with hepatitis was distributed by the Children's Hospital of Eastern Ontario. In at least one case, a patient was not notified of the recall by the hospital's blood bank or the hemophilia clinic. By the time the family heard of the recall, two weeks late, the patient had infused with the suspect product several times. "Even though no signs of hepatitis are apparent, the son . . . has undergone substantial emotional upset as a result of this lack of communication," a Hemophilia Society employee complained to Dr. Roslyn Herst of the Red Cross's Toronto Centre. At the time, Herst was also a medical advisor to the Hemophilia Society.

In this case, indications were that the Red Cross Blood Transfusion Service had acted properly in the recall, but the hospital was blamed for failing to follow through. Jo-Anne Harper, the official, called upon the society's medical advisors to draw up recommendations with respect to blood product recalls and how they should be carried out once hospitals had been informed by the Red Cross. "I'm sure you will concur on the seriousness of this matter. Recalls must be 100 per cent effective, especially when the alternative could be devastating to an individual and his health," Harper wrote.

Herst acted promptly, within a month drawing up a plan for user notification of a problem, and suggesting a nationally consistent notice be distributed with "wording appropriate to a non-medical person." A notice reminding the hospital blood banks of their responsibilities should be sent out before a recall occurs, Herst proposed.

Herst's draft notice said information must reach patients using home-care supplies quickly, especially in cases of recall. "The blood bank must telephone and/or mail the notices to these individuals. A hospital-based hemophilia program may assist with communications but it is the responsibility of the hospital blood bank, to whom the Red Cross issued the products, to ensure that the necessary information is disseminated," she wrote.

Herst's advice seemed sound enough, but the critical national recall necessary in the summer of 1985, when the old non-heat-treated product was to be returned, was badly botched. Bob O'Neill, then Ontario chapter director for the Canadian Hemophilia Society, says many patients didn't know of the recalls.

The Red Cross sent out notices to all hospitals around the end of June and early July 1985, Stephen Vick says. Non-heated concentrates were pulled back from the regional centres. At the Toronto centre, Herst avoided the charged meaning of the various levels of recall and asked for a "return" of any non-heated stock after July 1. Apparently some hospitals did not follow through — many hemophiliacs say they don't remember being contacted.

James Kreppner is one of those hemophiliacs who never heard the whistle blow. "No one ever called me and asked me to return non-heat-treated product." Kreppner told the Krever inquiry in 1994 that no one informed him not to use the old concentrates, either. It was never drawn to his attention. The Toronto lawyer says he didn't know there was a recall; in fact, he had come across some of the old product when he cleaned a room in his mother's house only two years ago. Kreppner was not alone.

It wasn't just home supplies that were forgotten. Johanne Decarie, her husband, Bill, and their young daughter, Billy Jo, are poignant proof that non-heat-treated, contaminated blood products continued to be used after the July 1985 deadline. In the case of this family from Rockland, Ontario, the offending concentrates were administered in a hospital, the Ottawa General.

Johanne — who is not a hemophiliac — had suffered a stroke in August 1985 when she gave birth to twins. She was transfused with Factor IX on several occasions between August 11 and 15. The hospital admitted in a letter sent in the summer of 1994 that the first of the transfused concentrates was contaminated. In fact, Johanne received five vials from the same lot that week — all of them probably contaminated.

Unaware that she was infected, Johanne transmitted the virus to

Bill. And later, despite the use of condoms, Johanne conceived Billy Jo. Now, because someone was asleep at the switch at the hospital, all three are HIV-positive. Bill and Johanne have become very active in the blood-infected community in Eastern Ontario.

"There was definitely not an adequate recall program," O'Neill says. "It was not efficient nor effective. The Red Cross has to account for that. But hemophiliac families have to account for that, too." O'Neill described how families had been stockpiling products and sharing supplies with cousins and other relatives. Often, bleed sheets were not kept. O'Neill says he did a survey which revealed that only a minority of hemophiliacs were sending in their record sheets to clinics.

"There were threats by the clinics to take away home care, but they couldn't deny people health care. Hemophiliac families and the clinics have a lot of blame for the inadequate recalls," O'Neill says today. "But the whole thing wasn't organized. The Red Cross would notify the hospital blood banks and feel their job was done. The Red Cross never really required records from the blood banks."

The gaps in the recall, for whatever reason, were dangerous. There were reports of non-heat-treated products still being in people's homes until well into 1986.

From our own family's experience, we know that recalls can fall short. In 1987, after some late infections among hemophiliacs in Western Canada, the Red Cross recalled sixty-seven lots of concentrates made by Cutter and Armour. Our son, David, had been sent products from one of those lots by the British Columbia Red Cross centre while visiting relatives. Two cousins who received the same concentrates received recall notices in late 1987 or early 1988. Although we could have been easily tracked down, we didn't even know that David had received recalled product until March 1994.

The lot that our son had received at that time, Cutter Commercial product No. 50P020, was raised at the Krever inquiry as an example of a recall failure. A memo had been received at the Newfoundland centre in late February 1987, but in November that year the same lot was listed again. "Would you agree that was not a sufficiently rapid response?" Dr. Huntsman was asked by the Krever inquiry. "Yes," he replied, "but it could be the responder who was at fault."

With heat treatment of blood products, one part of the protective shield against AIDS was believed to be in place. But some still had misgivings about the heat processing of blood products. What if it didn't work? There was another way to protect the recipients of blood products, and that was to stop the virus that caused AIDS from getting into the system in the first place. There were two elements to that preventative barrier: the effective screening of collected blood for deadly viruses and the exclusion, voluntary or otherwise, of high-risk donors. As with the heat-treatment process, both of these measures were adopted slowly and half-heartedly.

In July 1983, a blood bank at California's Stanford University began screening donors by measuring the ratio of cells known as helper and suppressor cells. Other tests were based upon the observation that the same groups of patients who were at risk for AIDS were also at risk for hepatitis B. Screen out those donors who had hepatitis B, and you might coincidentally catch those who carried the causative virus for AIDS. This method of identifying high-risk individuals was known as "surrogate testing." Officials at Stanford believe this testing may have prevented fifty to a hundred people at their blood bank from being infected with bad blood.

The connection between AIDS and hepatitis B had often been pointed out. It was known, for instance, that 85 per cent of severe Canadian hemophiliacs had evidence of exposure to hepatitis B. At the time, it was also known that 88 per cent of gay men with AIDS had hepatitis B antibodies, as well as 100 per cent of drug abusers with AIDS. This did not mean they were infectious with hepatitis B but simply that they had at some point come in contact with the virus and produced antibodies. Dr. Chris Tsoukas of Montreal remarked on the connection in April 1984. "The epidemiologic features of AIDS are strikingly like that of hepatitis B. It would certainly follow that another viral agent could be transferred in a similar fashion."

This information did not sink in with those who had hands-on control of the blood system. One former senior staff member of the Red Cross felt surrogate testing was better than nothing, but that virologists in the federal government regulatory structure would be better equipped to make that judgment. "We felt the push should be coming from the Laboratory Centre for Disease Control," the former employee says.

Dr. Gail Rock, then medical director at the Red Cross Ottawa centre, says she had an open argument with the agency's deputy national director of blood services, Dr. Martin Davey, over surrogate testing. Davey said the test was not worth the money. "It was clear to me at that point in time that this person was denying the medical evidence that was there," Rock told the Commons sub-committee in 1993. "The party line was AIDS was not transmitted through blood," she told me later. An American doctor expressed astonishment that Canada was not doing tests. "Canadians are really stupid to think AIDS stops at the border," she recalls him saying.

There was resistance to surrogate testing in the United States, where blood product manufacturers had been reluctant to proceed. A Cutter memo of late 1983 notes that representatives of four major companies decided to study the issue of testing "as a delaying tactic."

By mid-1984, a test had been developed that zeroed in on the HIV antibodies. Many experts harboured doubts about its accuracy because there were many false positive results — it had been described as "sensitive but non-specific." But the test's proponents argued there was now an effective way of screening blood donations and stopping the potential threat of new contamination entering the system. Later versions were markedly more accurate.

The method was known as the enzyme-linked immunosorbent assay, shortened to ELISA. It relied upon the appearance of antibodies in the human body when it is attacked by foreign agents. These antibodies normally kill or neutralize the invader and, once established, remain in the body to fight off further attacks. The ELISA test was originally developed to identify other retroviruses, but in June 1984 the American government issued licences to six companies to modify the test to specifically screen for HIV antibodies.

American blood banks started widespread clinical trials in September 1984, the same month that it was reported that heat treatment of clotting factors would kill HIV. Meanwhile, Canada's Laboratory Centre for Disease Control had started its tests on blood samples from high-risk groups in the summer, following the visits to the United States by Michael O'Shaughnessy.

By early October 1984, the Canadian Red Cross knew ELISA was potentially suitable for large-scale testing but had concerns about the scientific accuracy. It also worried about "very serious psycho-social implications" of rushing into widespread testing. One concern was that people who suspected they might be infected with HIV would dash to donate just to allay or confirm their fears. An American survey of donors suggested that 30 per cent would go to clinics to find out if they were HIV-positive. If there were many false negatives, it was argued, contamination of the blood supply might be worse than if nothing was done. The Red Cross didn't start evaluating the test kits from various manufacturers until the following February, and investigations continued until mid-May.

The results from the Red Cross and other laboratories suggested ELISA testing was both acceptably sensitive and specific. But there were also disturbing results. The preferred kit was made by Abbott Laboratories. Results of the testing revealed that of 3,000 samples from "random healthy donors," 15 were reactive to HIV. When a second test was done, 11 were reactive again and the other 4 were dismissed as "upjumpers." The repeat reactivity was 0.37 per cent of the 3,000 tests. This was not far behind rates already established in the United States.

This does not sound like a high danger rate. After all, it's only one positive in every three hundred donations. But when thousands of donations might be pooled to produce factor concentrates, the likelihood of infection soared. When severe hemophiliacs might inject vials of concentrate twice weekly, they would be playing Bleeders' Roulette.

There were other concerns. Those who still resisted the view that HIV was the precursor of AIDS (such as senior executives at the Red Cross), argued that a positive ELISA test might have no bearing on whether the donor could develop or pass on the fatal syndrome. Others said a negative test might mean nothing. HIV antibodies could develop at a later date after the donor was assumed to be free of infection, they suggested.

Other countries were less hesitant to introduce ELISA to their blood donors. Halfway around the world in New Zealand, the health ministry announced in November 1984 that all blood donations would be screened. South of the border, the National Hemophilia Foundation called for the testing of all blood donations in February 1985, just as the Canadian Red Cross was conducting clinical trials. In fact, nationwide ELISA testing in the United States began in early March on blood collected for American use. Some Canadian officials, defensive about the slower pace of ELISA adoption here, have argued that the American testing was phased in over the summer, but in fact the vast majority of donors were being checked within a month.

In Canada, Roger Perrault of the Red Cross said in May 1985 that there would be a transition period during which all incoming blood would be screened but untested stock would still be on the shelves. Delays were anticipated, he said, before all units issued could be screened. He also asserted that unscreened products would not be discarded, and screened products would not be given out preferentially to any user during the transition.

On the same day in March that the U.S. Food and Drug Administration waved the starter's flag for widespread ELISA testing, Canada's Task Force on AIDS-Associated Retrovirus Testing said it believed "a high proportion" of infectious blood and blood products would be eliminated from distribution if the kit was used. It cautioned, however, that the test would fail to detect a small number of infectious products. Meanwhile, the Canadian Red Cross asked for a delay in the use of screening tests until alternative sites were set up to provide for those who intended to use clinics to find out if they were HIV-positive rather than to donate blood.

This was a concern on both sides of the border. In the United States, some blood bankers wanted to delay notifying donors of the results of their tests. In Canada, the Red Cross wanted testing delayed for six months until facilities were established specifically for diagnostic tests, says a 1989 article by Sanda Rodgers in the *Ottawa Law Review*.

"The motives of those making the decision are not to be impugned," wrote Rodgers, then vice-dean of the law faculty at the University of Ottawa. "The concern was for the protection of the blood supply. Nonetheless, there are persons who may have been injured by infected blood during the six-month period when the implementation of testing was technologically feasible, but was not provided for reasons of a different order."

Pressure was building. Five days later, the National Advisory Committee on AIDS (NAC-AIDS) called for tests on all blood as soon as feasible. What prompted the call were results that showed 6 of every 1,000 tests of 60,000 blood samples in the United States had been shown to be HIV-positive in repeat tests. (The Canadian clinical tests had shown an infection rate of 3.7 of every 1,000 tests.) NAC-AIDS also urged the Red Cross to develop a plan by April 30 to implement screening of all blood donations. Six weeks later, medical advisors to the Canadian Hemophilia Society called for immediate institution of HIV testing.

Meanwhile, the Task Force on AIDS-Associated Retrovirus Testing came out in favour of the ELISA test as a good diagnostic test for HIV, complementing its screening utility. The group cited as evidence that ELISA had identified 2,000 positive tests in a cluster of samples from 9,000 high-risk donors.

Pressed into action, the Red Cross came up with a plan to start ELISA screening at all its blood transfusion centres by August 1, 1985, a month after the date recommended by the Hemophilia Society advisors. Blood collection centres would hire staff and sign a contract with the supplier in July, and training would begin.

The Red Cross proposal was accepted in June, but now came a delay in the approval of provincial government funding for the screening tests. The cost was estimated by the Red Cross at $2.4 million for 1985 and $5 million for 1986. After several delays, attributed largely to transition problems in Ontario's incoming government, final approval was granted by the Canadian Blood Committee on August 1. It would take another ten to twelve weeks before testing was fully implemented.

Dissidents who at the time worked for the Red Cross now question why that organization did not offer some of its substantial emergency or contingency money to bridge-fund the ELISA tests and get them started. The fund, then estimated at over $20 million, was tied up in income-generating investments, including short-term deposits, bonds, debentures, and stocks. Cashing some of it in might have imposed a cost on the Red Cross. "That was an occasion when the money was needed and it should have been immediately available," says Olaf Krassnitzky, who worked at the national Red Cross office at the time. The Red Cross board was asked to advance funds for the testing but chose not to. "At the time," says Krassnitzky, "I didn't think it was criminal, but I thought at least it was highly unethical." In 1994, that fund had an estimated worth of over $55 million. This is clear evidence that the Red Cross national office allowed other corporate priorities to submerge its responsibility for the blood system.

Some provinces were already wholeheartedly behind the screening test. Dr. Noel Buskard, the Red Cross medical director for British Columbia at the time, says his province could have been up and running the tests by September 1985. The kits had been given the okay in July and facilities were set. On the other hand, there were delays in training technicians who would conduct the tests. They were still being trained in late September. But British Columbia had given approval to the screening in June and was very supportive. In Alberta, according to public health official Bryce Larke, testing was started as early as September 19. If the kits had been available earlier in September, they could have been used. But money was needed for ELISA testing to begin.

Full implementation of the ELISA test in Canada finally began on November 1, eight months later than in the United States, and too late for many of those who suffered from the slow reaction of authorities.

Nationally, the Red Cross had done little to prepare its staff for the testing process. Bob O'Neill of the CHS reports a conversation with John Derrick in the summer of 1985, in which the Red Cross official said "once approval was received" the agency would start to train staff and set up at its seventeen collection centres to do the ELISA testing.

Bill Rudd, a former national president of the Canadian Hemophilia Society, expressed his consternation during the mid-summer of 1985: "We are not yet testing Canadian blood donations, and 50 per cent of our product is U.S.–source. This continues to be a major concern."

Rudd would not have known at that point how widespread ELISA testing was in the United States. However, he would have been aware of the delay of several months between the collection of blood and the distribution of American fractionated products in Canada. Furthermore, non-heat-treated American products were being imported until the spring of 1985 and were still being used in the summer. And non-screened products continued to be used in Canada for over two years after Rudd's complaint.

The snail's-pace decision-making was amply criticized. The *Medical Post,* in an editorial on August 20, 1985, called for an inquiry into the delay. The federal government could have put up interim funds and the Red Cross should have fought harder, the editorial argued. Three weeks later, on September 7, Hemophilia Ontario called for an inquiry into the ineffective steps taken to safeguard the blood supply against AIDS. Critics later charged that the Canadian Blood Committee was "an impediment to rapid decision-making in the face of a growing crisis."

One of the critics was Frank Terpstra, a hemophiliac and chair of the comprehensive care committee at CHS Ontario. He was also the representative of the Canadian Society of Clinical Chemists to the Canadian Blood Committee. In August 1985, Terpstra requested in writing an emergency meeting with Roger Perrault to discuss concerns about the safeguarding of blood against HIV. Perrault replied he would only talk to representatives from the national level.

In October, Terpstra commented on the protracted delay in the introduction of screening of blood donations by the ELISA test. "It could be argued that this delay put all Canadians to a significant and unnecessary risk of exposure to the AIDS virus and threatened the voluntary donor system as serious public concerns were raised during this period as to the safety of the blood supply."

Early in 1983, when internal alarms were being raised within the Red Cross about possible contamination of blood with the AIDS virus, regional medical directors were mulling over the idea of asking very specific questions to detect infected donors. The goal was to try to stop the suspected virus from tainting the blood supply. There were generally two camps within the organization. The regional officials wanted "reasonable" attempts to limit donations from individuals or groups of individuals who might be at high risk. It was suggested that donors who had suffered from night sweats, swollen glands, weight loss, or flu-like illness should be deferred for three months. This did not, of course, take into account the latency period in AIDS, when donors might feel they were well but in fact harboured the virus.

On the other side were the national officers, who felt blood collected from high-risk donors should not be singled out "at the moment." The argument was that, in Canada, donors got no economic advantage from donating blood and therefore could be trusted to be acting out of humanitarian instinct. One document quotes Dr. Martin Davey, assistant director of blood services, as saying no centre should be probing any more deeply than the basic question, Are you well? And "most definitely" no centre should be conducting their own diagnostic quiz.

In March, the Red Cross set up an ad hoc AIDS working group to examine ways of screening donors when they came to give blood. Considering the reluctance of many senior Red Cross officials to admit that AIDS was transmitted through blood, this was significant. A news release stated that while there was no evidence of AIDS transmission through blood, the Red Cross was asking that would-be donors in predetermined "risk groups" voluntarily exclude themselves. These risk groups were believed to be sexually promiscuous homosexuals, past and present intravenous drug users, and recent Haitian immigrants. The Red Cross said it would not question donors about their sexual preferences or national origin, and there was no general prohibition against gay men from donating. A second public announcement was issued in July, broadening the high-risk groups to include "sexually active gays or bisexuals with multiple partners," persons with AIDS or AIDS symptoms, and the sexual partners of those people. The release asserted it was the Red Cross's responsibility to do what is necessary to protect blood users from threats to health.

The announcements were hardly shouted from the rooftops. Red Cross officials apparently feared that if they were too explicit, they would scare off donors worried they could get AIDS in the process of giving blood. There was also concern that some rejected donors might raise a cry about human rights violations. In some regional centres, a laminated card listing the supposed risk groups was set out on the table where donors registered. Technicians would ask donors if any of the listed items applied to them. If donors answered yes, were not sure, or hesitated, they were asked to speak to a nurse on site.

Bill Mindell says Red Cross national officials had an "almost religious belief" that donors were altruistic. "They would not give something that was bad, or that they thought was bad. And they were terribly concerned about the protection of their donors. Not insulting the donors. Keeping the donors out of it. I have to say they honestly held those beliefs." Mindell says in all countries where donations are voluntary, the donor base is delicate and there is never enough blood.

Mindell recalls seeing a note from a Red Cross official saying if there was too much criticism, the donor base could drop by 30 per cent. "That was serious. There's only two ways to scare a hemophiliac: one is to tell them the blood is bad and the other is to tell them that there's no blood. And so we had to be very careful about what we did. We couldn't make outrageous and speculative statements."

David Page of the CHS says there was clearly concern in the Red Cross about the human rights of gay donors. "The gay groups were quite strong and they did have their own people within the Red Cross, so you had a legitimate concern not to surrender to the kind of homophobic accusations that were prevalent at the time. The problem is, we weren't dealing with human rights, we were dealing with public health, and if there had to be any erring on the side of caution, it was to be on the side of public health. That's where the Red Cross went wrong."

The Red Cross was already under fire for naming Haitians as a risk group, rather than specifying that it was Haitians engaged in specific sexual practices or drug use who were risky. And over-reaction was common at the time. Outrageous suggestions, such as the quarantine of AIDS patients and the banishing of gays to remote islands, had surfaced as the scare grew. National authorities chose to avoid asking specific medical questions to prospective blood donors. But the Red Cross working group on AIDS had been warned by Montreal lawyer Michael Worsoff as early as March 1983 that the organization had a "moral and legal obligation to protect the blood recipient above all."

Some regional centres, impatient with the timidity of the national office, took unofficial, unpublicized initiatives on their own to weed out questionable donors. In Vancouver, starting in the fall of 1982, nurses would make judgments about donors they encountered; if they had doubts, a green "destroy" tag was placed on the donation. Similar identification of doubtful donations was made at some other centres.

Noel Buskard defended this practice at the Krever inquiry. "The nurses at the clinic who had been collecting blood for five, ten, or fifteen years were extremely good at picking up high-risk donors who had read the card, had talked to the nurse, but still proceeded to donate," he said. Questions were raised about how objective this guessing game could be, but Buskard stood his ground. The reasons for tagging were not always subjective. When a donor had needle tracks, enlarged lymph nodes, tattoos, recent weight loss, or was chronically ill, the nurse would know that the blood was risky.

As 1983 wore on, the regional directors were virtually unanimous in arguing that questioning of donors about AIDS-related symptoms had to be more direct. In October 1983, the Red Cross working group on AIDS concluded that information on AIDS needed to be more specific and straightforward. Regional medical directors were frustrated with the tentative donor-screening policy adopted by the national Red Cross. But Perrault resisted these calls and reminded regional directors that the Red Cross was "not a democracy."

In terms of donor screening, Canada's efforts lagged behind those in the United States. Early in 1983, American blood banks had issued a caution against blood from donors in high-risk groups and were handing out brochures reinforcing the point. The National Hemophilia Foundation followed that up by asking the blood collectors to screen donors in an attempt to discourage donations from gay men. Similar advice came in March from the U.S. Public Health Service. This raised complaints from the gay community that blood collectors were not making a distinction between monogamous or sexually inactive gay men and those who had multiple partners, who were more likely to be high-risk donors.

When requests for screening were followed through, the result was a decline in the number of donors. Homosexual men had formed a disproportionately large segment of the blood-donating population in the United States. But many were not about to give blood if they had to disclose themselves to strangers. Tom Drees, a senior executive of Alpha Therapeutics, told the U.S. show *Frontline* that his company asked potential male donors face to face whether they had

had sex with other men. In the first week, said Drees, 308 said they had. Another 500 men just got up and walked out.

In New York, a more discreet system was worked out. After giving blood, donors could privately check off whether they wanted their donation to be used for research or to be transfused into patients. The process overcame the possibility that an infected donor might make a donation just to avoid being openly embarrassed. Several Canadian medical directors urged a similar system be adopted in Canada.

In April 1984, a year after high-risk donors in Canada were first advised through media releases not to give blood, the Red Cross produced its first information pamphlet for donors that contained information about AIDS. About 250,000 of those pamphlets were distributed over a three-month trial period. In some centres, the discarded pamphlets were recycled many times. That didn't stop busy collection centres from running out of the critical information. In April 1985, the manager of blood donor recruitment at the Toronto blood centre complained in a memo that there were often no pamphlets to hand out.

The high-risk groups listed in the pamphlet included gays or bisexual males with multiple partners, drug users, persons who visited or emigrated from "endemic" areas like Haiti and parts of Africa, and sexual partners of the above. "If after reading the pamphlets and the questionnaire you feel you shouldn't donate blood, you can indicate that to the nurse." There would be no obligation to say why you wanted to be deferred. In busy clinics, there was no way to be sure that a donor had actually read the pamphlet, of course, but the nurses still had the tag-and-destroy option.

August 1985 brought another national pamphlet which urged donors not to give blood if they were "active" homosexual or bisexual males. It also mentioned that a few hemophiliacs had developed AIDS because they were regular users of blood products made from the plasma of many donors.

Noel Buskard had become increasingly frustrated with the

national Red Cross. In November 1985, the B.C. region produced its own pamphlet, as did other regions. This one was much more explicit about high-risk donors. It asked for self-exclusion "if you are a male and have had sex with another male since 1977." Buskard said the previous references to "multiple" partners and "active" homosexuality were too vague. "We were unhappy with the questionnaire as it was. Finally we decided to go ahead and have our own questionnaires, despite national policy."

"Did we have the authority to do it? I guess we didn't. However, I would argue that my authority was to try and have the safest or the best blood system for B.C. That was my obligation."

Buskard made other innovations in British Columbia that spread across Canada. He introduced a donor signature requirement in 1987, in which donors had to indicate they had read the pamphlet. This was adopted in 1988 nationally. Another pamphlet in 1988 widened the restriction to gay men who had changed partners in the last six months.

Buskard claims these measures explain why the percentage of AIDS victims who were infected through blood transfusions in British Columbia is the lowest in Canada. (His figures excluded hemophiliacs who are HIV-infected.) He pointed out that in British Columbia there are 16 known blood-transfused victims, about 1 per cent of AIDS victims in the province, whereas in neighbouring Alberta, the figure is 24, about 4 per cent of the total persons with AIDS.

Meanwhile, in 1984, the American Red Cross toughened its restrictions, asking donors about lifestyle, risk factors, and the symptoms of AIDS. In Canada, those kinds of actions were not taken nationally until 1986. Oddly, no reference was ever made to spouses or sexual partners of hemophiliacs as potential high-risk donors, a frightening omission since this was a group of people very likely to make donations. The Krever inquiry heard of one Saskatchewan wife of a hemophiliac who became HIV-infected through her husband. She gave blood that was later traced to three blood-transfused victims.

As part of its implementation plan to introduce the ELISA test, the Red Cross said it would take steps to "reinforce the present process of informing donors about AIDS and persuading individuals at high risk not to donate." This practice would continue even after the testing was introduced.

Bob O'Neill, then an employee of Hemophilia Ontario, was a regular blood donor. In a memo written in early 1988, he reported that at his first donation in Toronto in 1985, there was nothing visible that discouraged high-risk donors from giving blood. "On the second occasion, I happened to notice a brochure on a table in the rest area following my donation." An inside page warned off high-risk donors. O'Neill wrote the Red Cross to suggest that donor self-exclusion information should be provided *before* blood is donated. O'Neill says he was told by Ron Rea, the Red Cross director of donor recruitment, that the brochures were deliberately kept low key.

The Hemophilia Society later noted that many Red Cross divisions had not distributed the pamphlets adequately. "During that critical period of the AIDS epidemic, hundreds of thousands of donors were not informed of the risk of contaminating the blood supply."

By 1986, however, New York–style self-exclusion had begun in some centres. Donors could check off whether their blood should be used for transfusions, used for testing only, or discarded. This was expanded nationally the following year.

Five years after the United States started requiring donors to complete a questionnaire before being interviewed by nurses, the Canadian Red Cross implemented a similar program. A full 10 to 12 per cent of prospective donors were excluded. "One can now evaluate how ineffective were the screening procedures in place prior to 1989," comments a chronology produced by the Hemophilia Society.

In late 1994, the Red Cross announced it would start using a more probing questionnaire, a decade too late for those who were already infected with HIV. The new format, taking effect in 1995, requires prospective donors to give responses to seventeen questions about AIDS, an increase from six questions on the previous form. And the questions will be asked verbally in private booths, because the theory is that people are more honest when they answer aloud.

If the Red Cross was slow off the mark to discourage high-risk donors, some members of the gay community were not. Physicians who treated gay men recognized a perilous situation — blood could carry the infectious agent that was mysteriously affecting many of their patients. Some influential gays, out of a mixture of altruism and fear that there would be a public backlash if contamination through blood became widespread, urged sexually active members of the gay community to stop donating blood. Their concern was well founded, especially in British Columbia where one provincial cabinet minister mused about the possibility of establishing a "leper colony" for people with AIDS.

Dr. Brian Willoughby, one of a group of seven Vancouver doctors with gay practices, told the Krever inquiry that he recalls a November 1982 article in *The Body Politic,* a gay and lesbian newspaper, that warned of an infectious agent in donated blood. A virus was believed the most likely cause of AIDS. Willoughby and colleagues urged that gay men reduce their number of sexual partners and stop giving blood.

Reinforcement for that stance came in February 1983, when Willoughby attended a meeting in Hawaii of the American Association of Physicians for Human Rights (AAPHR). Blood safety was on the agenda. It was announced that gays in San Francisco were being discouraged from giving blood. The AAPHR position was that gays who had had only one partner for the last ten years, or who were not sexually active, should not be excluded from donating. That was adopted as the "unofficial" policy of the Vancouver physicians and AIDS Vancouver early in 1983. The U.S. controversy at the time spilled over into Canada. Some gay activists refused to believe HIV could be passed on through blood and complained that restrictions were discriminatory. Some hemophiliacs wanted all gay men barred from making donations.

Willoughby went on record in a newspaper article in March 1983. "Gays who are sexually active shouldn't give blood. Instead, they should find a lesbian to take their place as blood donors."

There were nuances in the AAPHR position that might be too sophisticated for the local community, Willoughby told the Krever inquiry. "We were wiser to err on the side of caution by advising all gay men not to give blood."

Meanwhile, others were pursuing the idea of the so-called Sisters in Blood, based on the notion that after nuns, lesbians were the identifiable group least likely to be infected with AIDS. Noah Stewart, a founding member of AIDS Vancouver, was one of those who contacted a "sister" and asked her to take his place in making blood donations. To his knowledge, she is still giving blood today.

"We thought it would be worthwhile, because we felt that gay men should remove themselves as blood donors voluntarily," Stewart told the inquiry. "We had concerns that would cause problems in that the rate of blood donation would go down and perhaps blood wouldn't be available for people who needed it. So, we wanted to try to replace the blood that we were removing by blood which had no possibility of transmissible disease. We contemplated the idea that each gay man should ask a lesbian to donate blood on his behalf."

There's no indication that this ever became a widespread practice, but it reveals a level of concern and public-spiritedness that often wasn't evident in other circles. The Red Cross medical director in St. John's, Newfoundland, recalled a meeting with gay community leaders in 1983 in which they agreed to urge their members not to give blood until the transmission of AIDS had been clarified. But these commitments may not have reached bisexual men who did not consider themselves gay. In some cases the Red Cross was lax in making contact. In Montreal, for instance, there was no Red Cross representative on the local AIDS committee's panel of medical experts until 1986, despite an invitation made three years earlier. The Red Cross medical director in Montreal at the time has said that he was prevented by the national office from taking the initiative.

This lack of communication may have been the reason for some startling decisions by the Red Cross. In the spring of 1985, when HIV infection in the blood supply was peaking, the organization aggressively pursued blood donations by setting up a permanent clinic in Montreal's so-called Gay Village. That clinic was closed in 1986 after it was found that a quarter of the contaminated donations identified in Canada had been collected there.

ED KUBIN

"Have you ever experienced pain?"

It's a discomforting question that Ed Kubin asks, but not an idle one, coming from a man who has had his right leg amputated after infection and who has wrestled with death on several occasions.

Kubin, a hemophiliac who lives in a converted mobile home in Lorette, Manitoba, just outside Winnipeg, was close to financial ruin after becoming infected with HIV through contaminated Factor VIII concentrate. Even if he had dodged the bullet that struck so many severe hemophiliacs, the virus would have taken a heavy toll on his life. His younger brother Barry, also a hemophiliac, died of AIDS in 1991.

Kubin once put in fourteen-hour work days as a financial controller, earning a comfortable living. He blames HIV infection for the breakup of his marriage and his current state of impoverishment. Active in the Canadian Hemophilia Society for years, Kubin is credited with having started the push by hemophiliacs and the blood-transfused for compensation from governments. He is a proud man of angry words and dramatic gestures — characteristics that have won him admirers but also incurred enmity.

"I no longer have my job. I no longer have my family. I no longer have any money. This place here, I had to take on a boarder because I can't afford it. I haven't a clue what I'll do. I will be damned if I will go on welfare and become a charity case," he says firmly.

Kubin says it used to take all his tolerance of pain to get himself going in the morning.

"I had an extremely demanding lifestyle, four children (three girls and a boy), two knees that were shot, a really stressful job, and I was deeply involved in the Society. It got to the point where the pain was so bad I had to go on methadone and I took so much of that stuff that I was falling asleep and I would wake up screaming in pain. The nurse would say, 'How can you be in pain when you're falling asleep from the methadone!' I tell you, I *was*.

"I put up with that pain and I achieved above average income and lifestyle for my family, despite it. For me to go on welfare would be an insult of such immense proportions that I could not accept it."

When Ed Kubin talks about his brother and his mother, his voice — so often harsh — dramatically changes tone. It becomes almost tender.

"My brother Barry and my mother were both shoppers," he says. "You'd take an ox cart to get me into a shopping mall, but my brother was a 'Mallie.' He loved to shop, and so did my mother. They'd run into each other at the St. Vital Mall and sit and have a coffee and chat. My brother was one of those people who would have a list and he'd say, 'Ma, I've got to get going. I've got all these things to do.' And so he'd thunder off.

"After he died, mother would go to the mall looking for my brother. I'd phone her up and she'd say, 'Not too good today. I went to the mall and didn't see Barry.'

"Then, one day I called and she said, 'Not too good. I went to the mall, but this time I saw Barry and I went running after him, and when I got to him, it was somebody else.'

"She died about a year after him, in 1992. They are buried side by side, and I really think she died of a broken heart.

"When my brother died, it really upset me. But when my mother died, I was at peace. I was happy because I knew she was with my brother and that's where she wanted to be. She couldn't stand his loss. She couldn't come to grips with it, and it was driving her crazy. In my mind, her dying was a blessing."

Ed Kubin is direct and blunt. If he thinks you are spouting bullshit, he won't spare your feelings. If he is angry, he won't hold it back. That directness makes some shudder in the hierarchy of a group as historically moderate and dependent on the Red Cross and doctors as the Canadian Hemophilia Society, which Kubin once served as national secretary. His illness has not stopped him from speaking out. Indeed, much of what Kubin says sums up what many hemophiliacs and blood-transfused people firmly believe but are too polite or timid to say aloud.

"I am bitter about the treatment we have received from the governments, the way the Red Cross says their involvement was minimal. I have given a lot of thought to getting even with those sons of bitches, because they are enjoying prestige in the community, they have fancy incomes, they are looking forward to phenomenal retirement packages, and what have I got to look forward to? To me, if you knowingly cause the untimely, preventable death of an individual, you are guilty of murder, or at least criminal negligence. That's the way these people — the doctors, the Red Cross, the government officials — should be treated. Not one of those people will ever, ever pay anything for what they have done to us. They have totally destroyed us, and they have no compassion. They are not the least bit sorry."

When he becomes really ill with AIDS, Kubin will get into his truck, say goodbye to his children, now age fourteen to twenty-one, and head to the mountains where he finds joy, serenity, and peace.

"That's what I will do," he asserts. He takes a small object from his pocket and hands it across the side table. "I carry this with me." I gaze at it stunned, unable to speak.

"When I have no money and I can't do anything, that's the bullet that will end my life."

Chapter 9

THE HORROR UNFOLDS

"Where is the justice in the taking of a person's life by the people who are responsible for the safety of the blood products?"

PARENTS OF AN HIV-INFECTED HEMOPHILIAC, 1988.

Elaine Woloschuk, later to lead the Canadian Hemophilia Society into its battle for AIDS compensation, remembers being at an Ontario board meeting when another member made a frightening declaration.

"What we have feared has come to pass," he said. The first Ontario hemophiliac with AIDS-related complications had died.

"It wasn't classified as a death from AIDS," she recalls today. "People were very secretive, they camouflaged it. But it was Bill Mindell's view that the death had been from AIDS."

Mindell's memory is of a panic that started to set in. Studies at the time were starting to reveal very widespread HIV antibody contamination of hemophiliac populations.

"It was at this point I remember that I suddenly woke up to this thing and I realized: This is a horror story. Sometime between the summer and fall of '84 I just remember being terrified, because this was going to be a holocaust. They were all going to die. And it was on the skimpy evidence that I think everybody else had at that point."

A degree of fear had already hit many hemophiliacs, and in some cases the people they associated with. There was shock, denial, and a recognition in some quarters that other persons who used blood products might be infected, too. Even so, several years later

Hemophilia Society leaders received complaints from hemophiliacs who wanted AIDS and hemophilia issues kept completely distinct. They objected to being lumped together in the public consciousness with infected gays and drug users.

Mindell recalls the resistance to the subject of AIDS among hemophiliacs. The Hemophilia Society was largely run by two-parent traditional families at that point. "They just didn't relate to this stuff, nor did they want to be associated with it. They really didn't want to talk about it," he says.

Jo-Anne Harper, the Ontario coordinator in 1983, wanted to start an AIDS committee, Mindell remembers, and she clashed on the issue with Ed Gurney, then the CHS executive director. "There was a lot of opposition to that, but somehow we started it anyway. People were intimidated by [the] national [CHS]." Harper, Mindell, and a few others in Ontario got the AIDS committee going.

In January 1984, Mindell — along with two representatives of the AIDS Committee of Toronto — met with Ontario Health Minister Keith Norton. Mindell pointed out that many hemophiliacs were then living in fear of AIDS.

"They have fear of their treatments, they fear for their families — will wives or loved ones get AIDS from sexual or other relations?" says a note from that meeting. "Others have begun to fear hemophiliacs because of uncertainty and ignorance surrounding AIDS. Discrimination in the workplace and in living accommodations is entirely possible as it is with other groups; among children in school it may be unique."

Parents, too, felt guilt. They had often overseen the injections. Perhaps they had administered the contaminated products to their children, or handed them over to be injected. In one dramatic case before the Krever inquiry, a Toronto nurse testified she felt terrible guilt that she might have "hung" the unit that infected her mother, who had been admitted to the Wellesley Hospital after a brain aneurysm. An anguished parent of a hemophiliac could be left guessing which one of many units had been the fatal one.

Hemophilia Society leaders pointed out that their members were the only ones in high-risk groups who could not alter their behaviour to head off the horrible disease. Indeed, the fear of contracting AIDS through blood products was itself life-threatening if hemophiliacs declined to treat their bleeds.

News from the United States was not reassuring. The case of Ryan White, a young hemophiliac who was forced to change schools because of public hostility, was emerging. There were tales of homes being fire-bombed and spray-painted by vandals.

The spouses of infected hemophiliacs were being provided with erroneous and dangerous advice, if they were getting any at all. In February 1984, the National Hemophilia Foundation in the United States said the risk of heterosexual transmission of HIV by hemophiliacs was "truly remote." Some wives of hemophiliacs say doctors were telling them they were likely immune to the virus. The result was that many spouses became infected.

Bob Pedersen, who became national CHS president in the spring of 1986, says the society failed to provide adequate information to spouses. "We were told that this was an area of medical confidence. I think the CHS had an obligation to spouses of hemophiliacs, but we did not transgress the prerogative of our medical community to the point of giving confidential information."

Two Canadians who used blood products had died of AIDS-related illnesses in 1983, and the spread of the disease was continuing apace. Most doctors were still urging hemophiliacs not to modify their treatment, arguing that bleeding was still their dominant cause of death. Today's statistics show that was quickly changing: of 255 known Canadian hemophiliacs who died between 1980 and 1993, about 65 per cent (or 189) had AIDS-related deaths resulting from infection by tainted blood. Only 23, or 9 per cent, died from bleeds. Another 15 died of liver failure, 13 in accidents, and 15 of "unknown" causes. Remember, too, that in the first three years of that period, there were no deaths established as AIDS-related.

Mindell points out that euphemisms abounded in the hemophilia community. Medical advisors suggested until more was known about HIV transmission, hemophiliacs should delay having families. The word "condom" wasn't mentioned, but some doctors and nurses were presumably more explicit.

"There were other euphemisms," Mindell says. "Like, if you got pregnant you should discuss this with your doctor. That was a euphemism for abortion. These were individual decisions, and they're best not dealt with by scaring the whole population."

The biggest problem was dealing with small children. It was dangerous to send kids off to school without telling teachers and other school authorities that they were hemophiliacs. And when that information was disclosed, difficulties could arise.

Mindell, as a public health official, heard some of the cases of discrimination at his job in late 1984. "I had, at one point, grave misgivings that the public health system wasn't going to hold up under all of this, that they were going to cave in to some of the things that our law has prevented us from doing, like breaking confidentiality."

When testing of blood donations began, one Ontario medical officer contacted the Hemophilia Ontario office and asked for names of hemophiliacs in his jurisdiction who were HIV-positive. "It's confidential information, and he had no right to get it under those circumstances.

"Another was a high-profile medical officer who got caught in a meeting with a school board and eventually said he would reveal to the school board the names of all individuals in the schools who were HIV-positive. He got publicly caught in that one. My interpretation was it was a violation of our law."

Mindell was smack in the middle of another instance. One fact sheet he had worked on asked: "Will school officials be told about HIV-positive kids in the school?" The answer was no, followed by an explanation that it was provincial policy and law. The sheet was attacked in the *Toronto Sun* and no one from the Health Ministry would defend it. "I thought, my God, if nothing else, officials should be defending their own laws! That decision was driven entirely politically. They were just fearful of the gay community and of backlash from the non-gay community.

"Nothing in this disease was ever treated in the way we treated everything else. This was a time when people needed to be strong. And they weren't."

Denise Orieux, the mother of two grown hemophiliac sons, remembers driving from Toronto to a meeting in Montreal in 1984 with another woman whose son had been diagnosed HIV-positive. The other woman wanted to talk with Frank Schnabel, the Montrealer who founded the World Federation of Hemophilia.

Schnabel listened to the woman's descriptions of her son's illness. "The doctors will say he doesn't have AIDS," he told her. "But of course he has AIDS!" The son died the next year.

Denise, who says she was once the most trusting individual, made the rounds of the meeting room and asked the doctors in attendance what they thought about the connection between HIV and AIDS. The doctors were saying everything was fine.

"Every single doctor there said, 'Well, even if they're HIV-positive, it doesn't work the same on hemophiliacs. They take so much stuff [in their veins], they've got a kind of inhibitor towards it.'

"I said, Bullshit!"

Orieux says that Donald Francis, then at the Centers for Disease Control in Atlanta, has said there is no place on earth where the doctors could have got that information. It was the silliest thing he had ever heard.

"It was an absolute lie," she says today. "I think all of a sudden it hit them: my God, what have we done?"

As time passed, evidence that HIV was indeed the precursor to AIDS mounted. The group of severe hemophilia A patients that Chris Tsoukas, Hanna Strawczynski, and colleagues at the Montreal General

Hospital had started monitoring in the summer of 1982 showed progressive deterioration.

Initially, they were all healthy and none had clinical signs of AIDS, although two-thirds of the 34 patients had "evidence of cellular immune dysfunction." In 1982, 60 per cent were HIV-positive; by 1984 that seropositivity had risen to 97 per cent. By 1987, nearly 90 per cent of the group were showing clinical signs of HIV, 52 per cent had AIDS or "AIDS-related syndromes," three had died of AIDS, and one was ill of *Pneumocystis carinii* pneumonia.

The authors concluded that the majority of HIV-positive hemophiliacs would develop severe HIV disease within five years after exposure to the virus and all would display "progressive and significant deterioration."

Figures from the Federal Centre for AIDS in mid-1988, although clearly incomplete, reveal the sudden shock as detected infections from blood products rose. Two of the eighty-six listed infections were diagnosed in 1982, and one each in 1983 and 1984. By 1985, the number jumped to eighteen, in 1986 it was twenty-seven, and in 1987 there were thirty. With one startling exception — an Edmonton man who died of infection with cytomegalovirus in 1980, the others had been diagnosed in 1988. The listed victims ranged from a six-month-old baby girl from Montreal who died of pneumonia, to the Edmonton man who was eighty.

By the spring of 1985, it was "mathematically certain" — in the words of one Red Cross medical director — that Factor VIII concentrates made from large donor pools of untested blood were HIV-contaminated. This applied whether the product came from the United States or from Canada, although the amounts of virus in the Canadian concentrates might have been less.

Furthermore, the danger had multiplied many times for non-hemophiliac blood users, too. A report by the federal Laboratory Centre for Disease Control (LCDC), which was released in August 1994, estimated the risk of HIV infection in blood transfusions was as much as twenty-five to thirty-five times higher in 1985 than in

1978. A patient undergoing major surgery in 1985, who might require between thirty and forty-nine units of blood, faced a risk of infection of close to one in a hundred.

The LCDC report, based on data compiled by Robert Remis and Robert Palmer, estimated that as many as 1,441 Canadians might have been infected during that period through blood transfusion. That is higher than previous estimates and more than triple the 419 persons who had been officially reported by 1994. Even their low estimate of 942 was more than double the reported numbers. Because many of these blood recipients were very ill at the time of their transfusions, it's believed that more than half died from non-AIDS causes. But Remis and Palmer estimated that as many as 245 persons, but probably about 100, might still be unaware they are HIV-positive, capable of infecting sexual partners.

Toronto and Montreal were especially risky places to have surgery in the mid-1980s. The LCDC report estimated as many as 511 people, but more likely about 407, had been infected through transfusions in Toronto, with a range of 220 to 337 infections in Montreal. Vancouver was third, with a high estimate of 146 and a mid-range of 116 cases. There were some stunning regional variations—Halifax had more transfusion infections than Edmonton, Ottawa, or Quebec City. Calgary's toll was triple that of its neighbour, Edmonton, a reversal of the infection rate among hemophiliacs, which reflects the greater use of cryoprecipitate in southern Alberta.

When the Canadian Hemophilia Society turned in 1988 to the federal government for financial help for the victims of the tragedy, a large number of those afflicted wrote moving letters describing how their lives had been shattered.

One couple who had lost a son they described as vibrant and caring spoke of the betrayal they felt. "Where is the justice in the taking of a person's life by the people who are responsible for the safety of the blood products? Instead of the lifeline, the blood products have become a killer."

A professional woman, who had moved with her husband and

daughter to a small town, wrote of the fear of being ostracized. As her husband's illness worsened, his business had declined and respect in the community had been lost. Her little girl would grow up never knowing what a wonderful father she had, the woman wrote. There would be no way to compensate for the pain, the grief, and the suffering.

A young man spoke of being emotionally drained. "I constantly fear the future and doubt the present."

Before the campaign for government assistance began, the Canadian Hemophilia Society and its medical advisors seemed to be drifting, unable to cope with the unfolding tragedy. The CHS 1986 annual report said the previous year was one of "accomplishments, growth, commitment, concerns, and focus." There is no tone of anger or urgency in this message, no indication that 1985 was also a year of increasing death. The society, at the executive level at least, was doing just as it was told. At the membership level, it was uninformed, passive, and apprehensive. Dependency upon the Red Cross, undue respect for doctors, and the arrogation of power by those two groups had robbed the society of its rightful role as a consumer advocate for hemophiliacs. There was a large body of opinion — perhaps the majority — that criticism of the Red Cross would backfire on hemophiliacs. Either the Red Cross would punish hemophiliacs for raising embarrassing questions about the quality of blood, or donors might stop giving the commodity that was so precious, or both.

When consumer activists did try to get action, they were put down by the Red Cross and the doctors. For far too long, hemophiliacs had been told by doctors and hospitals what to do. They had played down their condition because of discrimination. Now, confronted by a new peril that had a grave stigma attached, most seemed paralyzed and unable to express their concerns: fears about losing jobs, of shunning by friends and even relatives, even fears about being the targets of violent acts. These things had happened to others with HIV antibodies, they had heard, and could happen to them too.

Hemophiliacs had often been tested for HIV by their doctors

without their knowledge or consent. Frequently, the results of those tests had been withheld. Those doctors who had control over the lives of blood recipients seldom considered the notion that physicians would be more effective treaters if their patients were fully informed, and that patients might actually provide useful advice had they been asked what they thought.

The message from the medical advisors noted that clinics had to change priorities to respond to "the difficult management and counselling problems encountered" as a result of the spread of HIV.

The prime players in the drama didn't seem to have any alternatives, and leadership was lacking, Mindell says. The Red Cross wanted AIDS cases as definitive proof there was danger.

"The scientific criteria they wanted — they were always on to this scientific thing, you had to have proof — was AIDS cases. By the time you had AIDS cases, you were dealing with a death. No other disease starts out like that. They were patronizing and they were arrogant, and they didn't want other people messing around their system. We weren't appropriate. But I ask today, Where was the Health Protection Branch in all of this? Somebody should have had oversight," he says. "We just had a lot of Chamberlains around when we needed a Churchill. You needed somebody extraordinary up there."

Pedersen, who took over as CHS president in what some have described as "the coup," has written that 1986 was "the most difficult transition in Society management I could ever have imagined. . . . AIDS made the trip from a far-off threat to the monster in our living-room from which there was no hiding, no escape, ultimately not even denial. It was a vicious punch in the face at a time when simply managing the financially troubled organization seemed a Herculean task."

The year before, Pedersen had been Ontario president. He recalls Mindell arguing then that users of blood products had to be alerted and must start taking control of the supply. "To be honest, we didn't have a clear idea of what the risks were, but I think Bill understood that people were going to die from these blood products. I didn't have a clear understanding because I felt that [Mindell] was one authority and our medical group was another. And the medical group was saying, 'We don't know, we don't know.' "

The national office was floundering. About $500,000 had been sunk into an unusable computer system that had been intended to permit an instant exchange of research data and treatment information, enhancing the quality of treatment for hemophiliacs. The mainframe turned out not to be suitable, and the costs of training would have been horrendous. In the winter of 1986–87, the society had a debt in the order of $300,000 on a disposable income of $50,000.

Pedersen hastens to add that there were volunteers of exceptional quality, but the society was in crisis. "The real problem was not so much that the individuals involved were dysfunctional but that they lacked focus and they lacked a comprehension of the impending crisis. I'm not differentiating them from the new gang that came in, myself included. We were equally dysfunctional because of our newness. The difference was the determination to say: what the hell is going on?" A new brand of aggressiveness evident in Ontario was transferred to the national executive.

"The new group had no great sense of victory when we took over. We were somewhere between despair and determination. It didn't get better in that first year. The meetings were traumatic, painful."

Pedersen says the newcomers changed the national society into an advocacy instrument for hemophiliacs. "We advocated very vigorously for improved products, for safe products. And a lot of the credit has to go to Bill Mindell and his level of expertise and to David Page, and the whole area of catastrophe relief. And Ed Kubin saying, 'I'm going to hold you accountable. You better do it right, or I'm going to get my shotgun and I'm going to do it right.' When a guy says that to you, you tend to pay attention."

Inadequately heat-treated or unscreened clotting factors continued to show up for at least two years after the introduction of the heat-treated products and the ELISA test. Mindell was still writing about withdrawal of outdated and possibly dangerous products in early 1987. In 1986 and 1987 some products slipped through the safety net.

Armour, the fractionating company that in 1985 had been contracted by the Red Cross to supply a quarter of the first lot of heat-treated concentrates, revealed in June 1986 that some European clients had become HIV-infected after using products from unscreened plasma. None of the seroconversions had occurred in Canada and the infected concentrates had been withdrawn.

Still, Dr. Robert Card, then chairman of the medical and scientific advisors for the Hemophilia Society, wrote to the Red Cross calling for an urgent review. Card noted Armour was to get a significant share of the coming year's contract for Factor VIII.

He wanted the Red Cross to check the effectiveness of the company's heat-treating method and find out if the method used in the implicated lots was any different than for supplies dispersed in Canada.

By October 22, 1986, Martin Davey of the Red Cross declared that any concentrates made from unscreened plasma had been removed from the Canadian blood system. Five days later, Roslyn Herst, deputy medical director at Toronto's blood transfusion centre, wrote that all Armour concentrates used in Canada were made from screened plasma and had been heat-treated. "It is not the same type of product that possibly was implicated in the HIV seroconversions in the recent United Kingdom cases and it will continue to be distributed by the Canadian Red Cross." She added that the contaminated product had not been tested before it was fractionated.

The issue just would not die. By February 1987, Card was again phoning and writing Davey, then acting national director. It had been brought to Card's attention that a small amount of unscreened concentrate was still in circulation.

"In the discussions that took place in October 1986 regarding the safety of Armour Factor VIII, I had understood that there were no factor concentrates prepared from unscreened donors still in the system," Card wrote. "I realize now . . . that whereas there was no such material in the blood transfusion centres, in fact there was a small amount remaining in circulation, having already been issued."

Card went on to say there was evidence that a few hemophiliacs "throughout the world" had become HIV-positive after having used unscreened but heat-treated product from more than one manufacturer. "Because of this, I strongly believe that all factor concentrate that is currently in the system and has been prepared from blood donors who were not screened for the HIV antibody should be recalled." Medical advisors to the Hemophilia Society were unanimous on that point. The Red Cross would have to ensure that checks had been made with hospitals and individuals so that all the products would be returned.

"I realize that at this point in time such a recall may lead to anxiety and fear among some hemophiliacs, but that does not change the necessity," Card added. "I recognize that such a withdrawal would add extra expense to the system, but I firmly believe that this step must be taken."

Card's toughly worded letter drew a quick response. Three days later, Davey said the Red Cross would take "discreet steps" to withdraw any unscreened product that had been distributed. The federal regulator, the Bureau of Biologics, would be informed of Card's request. All Red Cross centres would be notified and told not to redistribute any returned product.

Davey asked that doctors try to avoid any "undue alarm" among their patients. "We would especially appreciate being able to complete the process without attention in the media!"

He also tried offering words of comfort. The Factor VIII suppliers for the Red Cross in 1987 would be Cutter and Connaught. "The supplementary purchases from Cutter are guaranteed to come from anti-HIV-negative plasma, and their heat-treated product has not been implicated in seroconversions."

The recall letter that went out to hospital blood banks in March 1987 identified the offending products as made by Cutter. "Although these products are considered safe and have not, to the best of our knowledge, been implicated in any cases of HIV seroconversion, we have agreed to replace any unscreened product with product that was produced from screened plasma," one letter said.

Mindell wrote on April 27, 1987, that the situation described in exchanges between Card and Davey was "unacceptable and inexcusable." The Blood Transfusion Service, he complained, had given assurances in October 1986 that there were "no longer any unscreened [for HIV] concentrates in the system." This had proven wrong. Indeed, some unscreened products had been distributed in Ontario as late as February 1987. For those donations to be unscreened, they would have had to have been collected twenty-two months earlier if they were U.S.–source products, or fifteen months if Canadian-sourced. "How is this permissible (or possible) in a system that requires six months from collection to distribution and which the CRC-BTS [Canadian Red Cross Blood Transfusion Service] has continuously told us has almost no slack because of the demand?" Mindell asked.

"The principle applied to the safety of blood products with respect to HIV all along has been that the products are safe until proven otherwise, i.e., until infections have occurred and are reported. Then the products are withdrawn, recalled, etc. Is it not time that we begin to err on the side of caution and insist on products that appear to be safer, or put it another way, to stop using our children as the miner's canary!"

In October 1987, the blood system was rocked by news that six hemophiliacs in British Columbia and one in Alberta had become HIV-positive after using inadequately processed Armour concentrates. The seroconversions had shown up unexpectedly in a survey. Dr. John Furesz, director of the Bureau of Biologics, confirmed that the new infections occurred in spite of supposedly adequate precautions by the manufacturers. Early in November, the Red Cross did a "voluntary recall" of all the lots of products used by the seven known victims in the previous two years. That amounted to sixty-seven lots of Cutter and Armour Factor VIII and IX.

Subsequent investigation narrowed the suspect products down to three lots of Armour Factor VIII. Armour had used a dry, "short-heat" process to kill HIV, heating it for thirty hours at 60 degrees Celsius. (Cutter's process was seventy-two hours at 68 degrees.)

Several prominent AIDS and hemophilia specialists did a study on the 1987 seroconversions, with the results published in the *Canadian Medical Association Journal* in 1990. They noted that 2,427 donors had contributed 4,248 units of blood to the pool from which the contaminated products were made. Seven of the donors were found to be HIV-positive when they gave blood again several months later. "This appeared not to be an unusual event," the authors reported, adding that control lots showed comparable rates of infection. "The challenge to product safety apparently lies in the donation of plasma shortly after HIV infection and before detectable antibodies are produced." It would be impossible to ensure that donor plasma would be totally free from virus, they said, so better means of destroying HIV were required than the short dry-heat process that had been used by Armour.

Furesz reported that the three Armour lots were considered unsafe and were recalled by the Canadian Red Cross on December 10, 1987. "The recall action ensured that the earlier voluntary withdrawal was complete."

But the late infections had cast doubts on the process used by Armour. Furesz said future products might be processed through new methods believed to be more effective in eliminating viruses.

In October 1987, the advisory sub-group to the Canadian Blood Committee met in Ottawa with one item on the agenda being new immunopurified Factor VIII. This product was cleaner, purer, had less extraneous proteins to which a hemophiliac might react, and was as safe as any on the market, Dr. Kaiser Ali, medical advisor to the Canadian Hemophilia Society, told the group. It was also expensive for the time, at 55 cents U.S. per unit. But manufacturers had spent millions investing in it and now wanted to know if it would be approved for use before they spent even more.

Hemophiliacs in the United States and Canada, mindful of the latest round of HIV infections arising from dry-heated concentrates, wanted a better product, either vapour heat-treated or so-called monoclonally purified. Ali said, given the toll taken on hemophiliacs to that time, the CHS would drop dry-heated products in favour of the newer versions. (By then, deaths among blood recipients from AIDS-related complications as reported to the Federal Centre for AIDS had risen from two in 1983 to eight in 1985, twenty in 1986, and twenty-two in 1987.)

Dr. Gerry Growe, the representative of the Canadian Hematology Society and Vancouver hemophilia specialist, pointed out that this was an especially sensitive time when there were still seroconversions to HIV from products that had been counted on as being safe. "We must be able to respond quickly to products with enhanced viral inactivation," said Growe, who collaborated in the investigation of Armour that was later published in the *Canadian Medical Association Journal.*

In 1988, a deal was arranged with suppliers to provide the newer generation of vapour-treated products. The last dry-heated concentrate was sent out in July 1988. The Red Cross declared at the October 1988 advisory group meeting that it would not again distribute the dry-heated material, except for super-heated product. But the older discredited concentrate was still being dispensed in some hospitals at that time. Dr. Blair Whittemore, the Red Cross representative at the meeting, said he hoped the dry-heated material was not being stockpiled "for a rainy day."

One result of the late infections was that it gave Canada a jump on much of the world in 1988 in securing the next generation of vapour-heated products. Canadian authorities were a month ahead of those in other countries. Unlike 1984–85, when Canada fell behind in the game, supplies had been obtained by the time worldwide shortages hit. Even though some ordered quantities were "shorted," there was sufficient supply. But there was tension because governments seemed reluctant to foot the bill.

Stephen Vick, who was the Red Cross blood services director at the time, says there was pressure in the United States to restrict export of the newer concentrates. In the United States, operations were cancelled or postponed, and hemophiliacs had to resort to conservative use of the product.

"In Canada," says Vick, "we had locked up sufficient supplies to get us through. In fact, we ran a sham. The Hemophilia Society and ourselves pretended as if there were shortages here. We even used the hemophilia newsletter to talk about conservation and all the rest, even though at no time did we have less than four months' supply. In the middle of it we had a call from the hemophilia society in Missouri begging us to send down product because they had heard we had some and they had none in the entire state. It was really very serious. It took a little over a year, and it was resolved because the companies were able to gear up and improve yield."

Vick says the Canadian Red Cross couldn't have responded to the appeal from Missouri in any case, because once a blood product is exported from the United States, it wouldn't be allowed back.

He also says the Red Cross took a chance, buying the new products on an interim basis in the fall of 1987 as news was surfacing about the late infections. The purchases were made before approval had been given by the government funding agency, the Canadian Blood Committee (CBC). "It wasn't until early in 1988 that we actually had formal approval to go ahead, and it was Bill Mindell who was instrumental in helping us get that approval by putting some pressure on the Ontario government. We had tens of millions of dollars on order, and nothing to substantiate it at all, except our good will and the hope the governments would kick it through.

"They were interesting times, I will tell you. I saw my career pass before my eyes a few times," says Vick.

The hurdle in 1988 was the Canadian Blood Committee. Despite news of the outbreak of new HIV infections in Western Canada, hemophiliacs and their doctors still had to battle the CBC to get the best-available concentrates produced by Cutter Laboratories. Hot-vapour treatment was believed to be the safest method. But the CBC, unconvinced of the additional benefit arising from that new product, was unwilling to pay $25 million more to buy the new breed of concentrates. The Hemophilia Society knew it faced a huge selling job for the more expensive products. But Vick and Brian McSheffrey of the Red Cross were onside, and the Society's leaders were firm. A CHS document at the time said: "We cannot allow any financial considerations to compromise the health of hemophiliacs."

The climate was edgy. Doctors who treated hemophiliacs spoke angrily about the need for a secure system. The advisory committee chairman, Wayne Sullivan, did not want to be rushed. Pedersen says Sullivan's position was alarming.

"Our medical community was justifiably upset with that," Pedersen recalls. "It was very clear, if the chairman of a committee was pushing hard for non-action, it would be very hard for members of that advisory group to have any influence."

Dr. Kaiser Ali wrote federal Health Minister Jake Epp in May 1988. There was a world shortage of concentrates, he noted. If governments did not act immediately to replace the second-rate products then being used, there would be more hemophiliacs exposed to the risk of AIDS and hepatitis, and health care costs would rise. Bob O'Neill, who was working for the CHS then, says that in early 1988, for the first time, the hematologists had unequivocally taken the side of the hemophiliacs.

Pedersen, speaking as a parent of hemophiliacs to a meeting of blood experts in 1988, applauded their support for the speedy acquisition of the new vapour-treated products: "We do not believe, however, that this type of decision has always been the case in the past." Pedersen said the experts must apply their best medical and scientific judgments to decide which products were safest, and that he trusted in their judgment. But he added: "We only ask that if you may be making an error, then err on the side of caution for the benefit of the patients. It should be considered acceptable if the only thing wasted this time was money."

A stroke of luck occurred at a world AIDS conference in Stockholm. Vick had told Mindell that a five-year contract for the new products was ready to go but was being blocked by the Ontario representative on the Canadian Blood Committee. Mindell had gone to the AIDS meeting and there he spotted Elinor Caplan, then Ontario health minister. He cornered Caplan and explained the situation. She phoned back to Toronto, and two weeks later the logjam was broken.

The outcome was that the Red Cross and Cutter agreed to a five-year contract to supply Koate-HP. In today's context, some would describe Koate-HP as an intermediate-purity, vapour-heated product, since succeeded by much better ultra-high-purity products.

The length and terms of that deal, since extended, were criticized by some Hemophilia Society leaders when superior concentrates became available. Bob O'Neill says the new products finally stopped the transmission of HIV through the concentrates. He says Vick and McSheffrey stuck their necks out because the Canadian Blood Committee did not like the Red Cross ordering the products before funding was approved.

"It was the best deal anywhere," maintains O'Neill. "Cutter was willing to give us a price cheaper than what they were charging in the United States. At the time it was the No. 1 product."

"Is he still alive?"

That is the saddest question a member of the hemophilia or blood-transfused communities can ask in the late 1980s and early 1990s. But if you haven't seen someone in a while, it becomes second nature to ask. The scandal of it is that this question is not asked about people in their seventies or eighties; it's about younger adults from their teens to their fifties. It is an appalling loss to Canadian society.

ALLISON BROWN

Allison Brown of Ottawa is a hemophiliac who says his young family was put at risk by a doctor he trusted and had gone to for seventeen years.

After Allison's wife, Grace, became pregnant, her obstetrician suggested she have her blood tested. "I was insulted," says Brown.

"I had been told I was negative." Still, he called the nurse at the Ottawa General's hemophilia clinic. "She said, 'I hate to tell you this over the phone, but you are not negative, you are positive.' That was my initial baptism."

Brown, originally from Sussex, New Brunswick, recalls going to his doctor two or three times in 1986 after his blood was taken for testing. The doctor said the tests were not back. The results seemed slow in coming. Finally, the doctor told him: "You're negative. Only bad news comes back fast."

Before Grace and Allison left Saint John for Ottawa, they went to the doctor to pick up a letter. "He made an unsolicited remark to Grace. 'Don't worry about Allison — he looks after himself well, and you'll have a long and happy life.'" The doctor would have known of Brown's status for a year.

"People have so much trouble asking doctors questions, and then when they do ask the right questions, they don't always get an honest answer," Brown says bitterly today. "He endangered my wife and child."

Brown says the doctor has contradicted his own comments. At the discovery for a lawsuit Brown brought against him, the doctor said he didn't break the news that Brown was HIV-positive because he had another hemophiliac patient who had given up on life when he'd been told — quit his job, gone on welfare, and stayed home all the time. Then later he said, "You must remember Allison was the first one in New Brunswick to be tested."

JIM SMYTH

Winnipeg hemophiliac Jim Smyth wasn't feeling up to par in the winter of 1983–84. He was getting married in February, so he went to his doctors for a check-up to make sure he was all right.

"They were all telling me I was fine, there was nothing wrong with me." But Smyth was bothered by the way he felt and kept pushing for answers. Finally, one of them said that he might have some viral infection but it would be like a cold and then pass.

"Don't worry about it. Go ahead, get married, have kids," Smyth says he was told. Three months after the marriage, he still wasn't feeling right. His wife suggested he go to her doctor.

"He just happened to work with a gay men's health clinic. And as soon as he saw me and heard my symptoms, he sent me to see Dr. Bob Brunham [an infectious diseases specialist]. He diagnosed it — that was mid-1984."

Smyth informed his hemophilia doctors and got an earful. "I went 'behind their backs,' they said. I had no right going to see another doctor. I got quite a chewing-out. I was shocked.

"They told me they knew about it, but they didn't want anything to be said about it at that point — it would cause a panic. I grabbed a handful of quarters and headed for the phone, and called a few of the other guys I knew. After I found out what Bob Brunham told me about — that it was infectious — I couldn't see leaving anybody without the knowledge. They could be infecting family members and so on. So I informed them."

JUSTIN MARCHE

Bill and Rita Marche of Newfoundland had trouble finding out about the status of their son, Justin, too. After Justin became infected, they read all they could about the disease and sent away for information. They learned about the role of T-cell counts as an indicator of the strength of the immune system, for example.

"We went to our doctor wanting to know where Justin stood, what his counts were, because that would give us an indication of whether the virus was progressing," says Rita. "He just wouldn't give us any information at all. He kept putting us off and saying we wouldn't understand it."

The couple, along with Rita's two hemophiliac brothers and their wives, then confronted the doctor and demanded he tell them what he knew. Rita says the doctor told them that when Justin's count reached the low point at which drug therapy was needed, they would be the first to know. But it didn't happen.

A trial came up for Ribavirin, a new drug. Only patients with T-cell counts between 500 and 800 could participate in the trial. Rita's two brothers had T-cell levels too low to allow their participation. In fact, they should have already been on the drug AZT.

"Obviously, they hadn't been notified," says Rita. "So they contacted us. We were living in Fredericton at the time. I took Justin to be tested there and his count was down to 16."

The New Brunswick doctor asked what Justin's T-cell levels were before, and Rita admitted she didn't know. The doctor in Fredericton was astonished. "Why don't you know? Didn't you ask?" And Rita replied, " 'Of course we've asked, we've been harassing our doctor.' He just could not believe it.

"We will never know, I suppose, if it would have made a difference, but Justin — very soon after that — began AIDS dementia. The only drug they've found that works is AZT, so you kind of feel that if he had been on it sooner, that it's maybe something that could have prevented, or lessened, or given him at least a bit of quality of life."

Chapter 10

NOTIFICATION FIASCO

"Contagious disease? What is he talking about?"

MARLENE FREISE, 1991

Marlene Freise's blood was contaminated by a transfusion in 1982. It was nine years before she discovered what had happened, and that was purely by chance.

Marlene and her husband, Jerald, had routine medicals done in 1991 when they applied for life insurance. When the word came from the insurance company that Marlene had been rejected because she had a contagious disease, they thought there had been a mistake.

Incredibly, the way was barred even when they tried to find out what this mysterious disease was. There was no explanation from the insurance agent; no one was available.

"So we were saying to ourselves: 'Contagious disease? What is he talking about?' This is totally out of the blue," says the Scotland-born Marlene, surrounded by the Oriental decor of her Toronto living-room.

"Then it dawned on me that he had done the AIDS test, and I knew what it had to be. I just knew it. And I was pretty much totally shocked. I never slept that night. You're crying your eyes out. You're dreaming about terrible stuff and you wake up and you're crying."

In the morning, Jerry tried to get word from the insurance agent. He was not in and Jerry was angry. "They left you with this big question mark in your life and nobody has the courtesy or the decency to let you know," Marlene adds.

The couple have two children and their daughter Whitney was born after Marlene was infected. This was the next concern. "Your thoughts are, Oh, my God, the kids are going to get taunted at school, and they're going to have no friends. So, you're feeling absolutely abandoned by anybody who has any knowledge of it or can give you any comfort. You don't want to tell a soul. You don't want to tell your family. Nobody."

"The ones you do call — like the Red Cross — they slam the door on you," says Jerry.

Marlene received the news in January 1991. It took until April before she could bear to get Whitney tested. "You know, you go through the questions: Well, what if I die before she dies? I just couldn't imagine this little three-year-old lying in a bed just absolutely devastated health-wise, and not having a mother there." When Whitney's test was finally done, it came back negative, which for Marlene emphasized her isolation.

The Freises were never notified by the Red Cross or any other agency that Marlene was at risk of infection. For blood-transfused victims, their experience was the rule rather than the exception.

Jerry and Marlene Freise became driving forces behind the so-called HIV-T group, representing many of those who have been infected by blood transfusions generally in the course of other treatments. They have also been a source of information for newly informed patients who don't know where to turn.

"We're finding people all the time," Jerry said in the fall of 1993. "We come from all cultural backgrounds, all kinds of socio-economic status. And I think, therefore, that we represent the general Canadian public on this issue. We are just a bunch of people who are impacted by this."

He listed some recent cases: "A lady who was infected found out through insurance. She has two young children, and she's going to have them tested. Another lady is a nurse in her early forties. She, too, has two young children. Her husband just tested negative. Another man has a nine-year-old son who was born premature. Got a bit of a 'top-up' as they used to call it — a teaspoon of blood to compensate for what they were taking out of him in blood samples. He was infected. For years he'd been getting asthma tests, this test and that test. Another lady has a nine-year-old girl who had symptoms and just got tested. The girl's dying already."

Freise says there should have been a national recall of blood, and a national notification program.

"A lot of people didn't know they had transfusions. They were out cold during the operation and didn't think of a transfusion. If it's a parent down at Sick Kids [Hospital for Sick Children in Toronto] during a cardiac operation, the last thing they would worry about is a transfusion. They are concerned about the cardiac condition. One parent asked his doctor and the doctor said, 'No, I don't think your daughter had a transfusion. One out of 100 chances.' And it turned out she did have a transfusion. It also turned out she was negative. But this is a problem. A lot of people don't know."

Freise's reading of the voluminous documents has led him to conclude there was a cover-up of massive proportions. "There was a massive involvement of the medical profession, including hospitals, doctors, nurses, but primarily the Red Cross, ministries of health — all governments, federal and provincial. They may find that they knew at various levels and degrees at various times what the problems were. But I don't think they will think of any excuse for the silence of the past nine years. I can't think of any excuse these people can have. Especially when you have government officials coming out and saying, as they did [about the infection rate among hemophiliacs], 'Oh, we all knew that.' Trouble was, they didn't tell anybody!"

Freise says today he is appalled at how the simple act of caring for people in Canadian society could become a contentious political issue. "I'm talking about the people who turned their faces from the knowledge of what was going on. Life went on normally at the surface, but there were people who knew . . . The horror of it is not dramatic. The horror is banal . . ."

One of the abysmal failures in the sordid story of contaminated blood is the lack of notification of the victims. Instead of getting down to the business of tracking recipients of bad blood, the buck was passed without consideration of people's lives. The Red Cross, sloughing off responsibility, said the onus was on hospitals or doctors to notify those at risk. Worse, when Red Cross officials were asked to help locate those who might have been infected, they jettisoned any humanitarian instinct and covered their backsides.

In one Ontario check, only 5 of 41 people who received contaminated blood through transfusions were ever contacted by authorities over periods of up to twelve years. And in a national survey done on November 1992, only 26 of 103 victims who replied had been tracked down through an official tracing system. The rest found out on their own. The system, if it can be described as that, seems to have failed most in Ontario and Quebec.

Poor hospital record-keeping and a mobile Canadian population are factors. Before 1984, many hospitals kept blood bank records for only six months to a year. And even when donors or recipients of risky blood have been identified, they may have moved without leaving a forwarding address. But the plain fact is that a significant effort in many cases just was not mounted.

If you are infected with an inevitably fatal disease like AIDS, how important is it to be told? The ill have a right to know why their health is deteriorating. The paternalism that still exists among some members of the medical professions has no place today. Knowledge of your illness allows you the opportunity to seek information on how to reduce the risk of the disease both to yourself and to others. It also allows the victim to choose treatment options to prolong life. In the case of a disease like AIDS, Dr. Alexander Klein told the Krever blood inquiry, you could be walking around with advanced symptoms without knowing what is wrong. "You're a walking time bomb," he added.

Jack McDonald was spurned by the Red Cross when he requested the agency's help in searching for the victims of tainted blood. He first wrote a letter to the humanitarian agency. Then, in the fall of 1989, the associate professor of social work at the University of Calgary stopped by Red Cross headquarters in Ottawa. McDonald wanted to know if the Red Cross would help identify persons infected through blood transfusions (other than hemophiliacs), determine their numbers, and sponsor a national support and education program. He got no response for several months. When McDonald followed up with another letter, he received a reply from the secretary-general at the time, George Weber, saying that on the advice of their lawyers, the Red Cross could not see its way clear to assist in any way. "The Red Cross was not interested in assisting with any efforts to provide support and information to this population," according to a report McDonald filed with the House of Commons in 1993. As astonishing as the reply was, McDonald said in an interview he wasn't surprised, from what he'd learned about the Red Cross.

He found little backing elsewhere, either. In January 1990, McDonald tested the waters at the Canadian AIDS Society, approaching the national executive director. "His response was less than encouraging," the report to the Commons says.

"So then I said, 'Well, I've got one more card — it's the Canadian Hemophilia Society.'" He wrote the CHS, and they replied they were supportive in principle as long as it didn't cost the cash-strapped society any money. The CHS agreed to apply to Health and Welfare Canada to fund a project designed by McDonald for blood-transfused victims.

Even after the study was completed — researchers had found 261 blood-transfused victims by October 1992, nearly half of whom had died — the message wasn't easy to get out. Both the journal of the Canadian Medical Association and the journal of the Canadian Public Health Association rejected an article on the findings.

Meanwhile, many doctors who had HIV-positive patients under their care for years were slipshod in breaking the news. Others seem to have been reluctant to disclose the information because of the stigma of AIDS and the fact that in the early years at least, treatment of the infection was non-existent. Then, after infection was made known, there were lapses in keeping patients and their families up-to-date. Even some hemophiliacs, who have regular clinic appointments for blood tests and are accustomed to bad news, found their doctors less than forthcoming.

Medical authorities were much concerned in 1985 with how to go about notifying the donors of contaminated blood. There was the fear that unless testing sites — other than the Red Cross collection centres — were set up, many people nervous about HIV and AIDS would rush to give blood solely to find out if they were infected. Since the screening tests of the day were imperfect, the blood supply could be put at greater risk if there were many "false negatives" among the donors. Less attention was paid to finding and warning the recipients. The search for infected donors was certainly a legitimate concern, but the process seems to have been very one-sided.

The National Advisory Committee on AIDS met May 15, 1985, shortly after the start of distribution of heat-treated blood products, but before the introduction in Canada of the ELISA screening test. Roger Perrault of the Red Cross moved that a conference be organized under authority of the Canadian Blood Committee to assess the impact of notifying donors of the results of HIV-antibody testing. He wanted a thorough examination of the sociological, ethical, legal, medical, and other facets. Among the subjects was the development of information for donors and for health-care workers to use when informing victims of their HIV status. The Red Cross, said Perrault, did not want to get into a donor-notification service until all the issues had been explored at the meeting. Eventually, he said, donor notification would be implemented by the Red Cross. Not everyone was happy with that promise of future action. Dr. R. G. Mathias of Vancouver, chair of the Task Force on HTLV-III Testing in Canada, "found it difficult to accept non-notification of donors and wished his objection to be recorded." He was a minority voice — eight of the ten NAC-AIDS members present voted in favour of the Red Cross position.

The question was then raised whether the conference should also discuss the impact of notification of recipients as well. "Considerable discussion took place as to whether the impact will be limited to 'donors' or whether 'recipients' could be included," according to minutes of the meeting. "Dr. Perrault felt that because the issue arose out of CRC [Canadian Red Cross] screening, that 'donors only' should be adhered to but he agreed that the wording of the motion could involve recipients. [Dr. J. Allen of the Centers for Disease Control in Atlanta] pointed out that the issues regarding recipients of reactive blood were very different from that of donors who produced it and agreed with Dr. Perrault that maybe the issue should be handled separately. A federal government lawyer indicated that, from a legal point of view, major concerns may be related to donors but there was a growing swell of additional concerns on the part of the recipients."

The motion was approved with only one abstention. Donors were included; recipients were not.

Over a year later, Perrault mentioned at a meeting of the Canadian Blood Committee that there were "major problems" in checking back on the blood components of donors who later test positive for the virus. This was because of the unavailability of blood-bank records beyond a couple of years and the variation in hospital record-keeping across the country. "He added that 450 recipients might be involved annually in any lookback procedure."

A legal action that gained national exposure was the suit against Dr. Stanley Bain of Toronto by Rochelle Pittman. Pittman's husband, a heart patient in his mid-fifties, received a transfusion during a coronary bypass in 1984. He was later tested and found to be HIV-positive. But Bain never warned the Pittmans. He assumed the couple were not having sex because of their age and his patient's condition. But Bain was wrong, and Rochelle became infected. Her husband died in 1990 without ever knowing he had AIDS.

"A month later I was informed he had tested positive for the AIDS virus," Rochelle Pittman told the Commons sub-committee on health issues. "I was shocked and terrified. My first thought was, Am I also infected? Six months later this fear was realized when I also tested HIV-positive."

In court testimony in November 1993, Bain said he didn't tell the Pittmans because the husband's heart was so weak he might have had a fatal attack. But because Bain failed to inform her or her husband, Rochelle now faces death from AIDS, too.

"I just feel that something needs to be done because the system hasn't worked properly," Pittman said in November 1992. "I think if my husband had known, he might well be alive today. He lived six years without any medical intervention in any way, and it just seems to me that nobody really cared."

The suit by Rochelle Pittman and her family against Bain, the Toronto Hospital, and the Canadian Red Cross Society was a pivotal case, watched closely by all those who had become HIV-infected through blood products. The family was awarded $515,000 and about $370,000 in legal costs by Judge Susan Lang in a judgment of over three hundred pages. The failure to notify the patient and his family bore heavily on the decision.

What's particularly striking is how poorly the system performed in this case. This was a relatively simple situation in which a single donor of the cryoprecipitate that was transfused into Kenneth Pittman in 1984 was identified as HIV-positive in January 1986. Yet it took nearly a year and a half for the Red Cross to inform the hospital of the infected blood product. It was close to two years later, in April 1989, that the hospital told Bain. And Bain had eleven months before Pittman's death to tell his patient but neglected to do so. Worse, he failed to tell Mrs. Pittman.

Judge Lang said it was clear Kenneth Pittman wanted to know what was wrong with him. "While information about one's bad health is clearly 'bad news,' a patient is entitled to know that is his or her prognosis, absent clear indication that he or she does not want to receive that news."

* * *

Dr. Roslyn Herst, medical director of the Red Cross Toronto Blood Centre, describes a complex process of identifying donors of infected blood that involved manual checks through hundreds or thousands of records to find out which hospitals might have received dangerous products. The process, known as a "lookback," could not be started unless a donor's HIV status became known, she said. Red Cross officials often cite a theoretical situation in which a one-time donor seroconverts after giving blood. In that case, there would likely be no way to identify the source of contaminated blood. "With a number of our earlier donors, we had no way of knowing their HIV status, and had no trigger to begin to look for which of our millions of transfusion recipients over the many years should be alerted to the fact they might be infected," Herst told the Commons subcommittee in the fall of 1992. "We did not have that trigger in all the cases, which may account for the perception that people who were infected by transfusion were not notified by the Red Cross because of some failing."

The first full lookback done by the Red Cross occurred in 1987, although a similar process was done as early as 1985 when there were proven transfusion links, Herst told the Krever inquiry.

Another way of identifying potential victims was if a transfusion recipient became infected. Checks could be made to see what specific blood units the person had received during an operation and then the numbers could be tracked back to narrow down other recipients and the donor. This is known in the trade as a "traceback," and the first one occurred in the summer of 1985. But Herst told the committee that the Red Cross did not know the recipient patients or doctors. "The trail gets picked up by the hospital at that point and they take it backward. If the recipient of the blood tests positive, it has nothing directly to do with the Red Cross."

Roger Perrault offered testimony similar to Herst's: "We can only act on that if the hospital brings it to our attention." He told the subcommittee that he had "vivid memories" of the problems involved in tracebacks. "One particular patient from Vancouver had received over three hundred units of blood from three hundred different people," Perrault recalled. "This was an elderly woman and we started systematically testing. I approved special budgets for that, because it cost us in excess of $20,000 just to track down. . . . " He hesitated, then continued: "We put a full-time nurse on that, to be able to track down the three hundred donors."

One might expect that the woman — and the three hundred donors, for that matter — would have thought it was well worth the $20,000 to track down the infected donor.

"In the tracking-down process," Perrault continued, "you can imagine the anguish of getting a phone call saying that your blood may have been involved in the contamination of a patient. Some people were helpful in coming forth and wanting to be tested. Some did not want to be tested. Others threatened to sue if we carried on the conversation. And others were untrackable."

Herst told the Krever inquiry that despite the computer age, tracking is still being done with difficulty and still involves a paper trail. "What we really need is a full integration of test results and past donations and issue records, and that full integration has not been achieved on computer." The Red Cross hoped to have its integrated system up and running in early 1995.

The Red Cross seems to have been excessively reserved in notifying infected donors in 1985. In March, Dr. Marlis Schroeder, medical director at the Winnipeg regional centre, told a group of hemophiliacs and medical colleagues that if a donor's blood tested positive, the donor would not be informed of the result.

"The blood product from that donor will be discarded. An aliquot of that blood will be frozen so that at a time, we don't know when, a confirmatory test is available, those samples would be thawed," she said. Schroeder suggested donors could be panicked by telling them they were HTLV-III positive, if there were no evidence of major problems with infection and they were "entirely healthy."

"So, I think in the interim that information will be kept totally confidential. When that donor returns to give another donation in three months, they will be retested and if they are again positive, a sample will be frozen and this will be continued until further information. I think it's going to cause major logistics problems at blood banks."

Schroeder was asked whether blood would be accepted from a donor on a second visit, if a previously positive donor tested negative on his return.

"It will be coded on computer," replied Schroeder, "and we will be able to identify the individual who is HTLV-positive and therefore will be able to follow up. There will be a method of identifying the donor. The information at the present time will be kept in the blood centre."

The Red Cross reluctance to notify HIV-infected donors was never more explicitly demonstrated than on October 16, 1985, when a statement was issued by national headquarters. Against the existing evidence, and despite the introduction of the ELISA screening test across Canada, the Red Cross expected four out of five reactive tests would be "false positives."

"The Red Cross considers it responsible to notify its donors only when we have a high degree of assurance that we have detected antibody to the AIDS-associated virus," said the statement. "We feel that notification when there is a very low probability of infection is unnecessary and prejudicial to our donors."

This timid stance in the face of danger to public safety was approved by J. McCrea, the acting secretary-general of the Red Cross; Dr. Martin Davey, assistant national director of the blood transfusion service; and Kenneth Mews, technical information officer with the Red Cross AIDS project.

While the information was being recorded, computer-coded, and held quietly by the Red Cross, one has to wonder how many identifiable donors were at large unknowingly infecting their sexual partners. The same day in 1992 that Roslyn Herst first testified before the Commons sub-committee, Robert St-Pierre, the Canadian Hemophilia Society's coordinator for people infected through transfusions, described the blood system as fragmented and marked by lack of communication.

"We have a system with many partners: the Red Cross with its donor files, which is crucial information for tracing people; we have the transfusing hospitals with the medical files; and we have the treating physicians," St-Pierre told the sub-committee. "There's no way to ensure that if I put in the information at one end, it'll come out the other end. And what we're looking for is, when you come out at the other end, the person who received the contaminated blood has been notified.

"We need a recommendation that will go out across Canada, telling the physicians that if their patients were blood-transfused between 1978 and 1986, they should get an HIV test. That should be a must."

Jack McDonald says he wasn't surprised when the Red Cross rejected his request that they help seek out those infected by blood transfusions. "My feeling was that they probably *wouldn't* cooperate."

The Red Cross may have reacted that way because of the fear of legal action. If more people transfused with tainted blood turned up, more suits might be launched.

McDonald says one official acknowledged the search was a Red Cross responsibility, but that the organization was immobilized by fear. "We can't act on our humanitarian responsibilities because of the fear this has elicited within the organization," McDonald recalls him saying.

McDonald explained in November that his social work experience helped him understand why his effort was spurned by the Red Cross. "My profession constantly works on diagnosing what is going on. For several years I had seen the Red Cross as an exceptionally insular organization, totally preoccupied with itself, totally top-down driven, and in a state of mass confusion. So when I saw it behaving the way it behaved, I said, 'What else can you expect?' That's what goes on there, and it wasn't a surprise, and I didn't waste a lot of energy over it. I guess I saw it as an establishment-oriented organization that had been a pillar of service for many years but was infiltrated by what I saw as exceptionally strong social statuses. And if you didn't belong to those social statuses, you didn't have any say in anything."

McDonald saw the medical directors at the Red Cross as some of the finest people he had met. But the society itself was "dysfunctional."

"My reaction was, I'm being patronized again so I won't waste any time with you. And really what I wanted was documentation that they wouldn't do anything," McDonald said in November 1993. "They've now put it on record they are not interested in this population or in helping them."

Now that many blood-transfused people in Canada have been identified, McDonald sees them working for an improved blood system. "The people who are fighting the fight are the people who should. There's been a real emergence of people who want to look at the blood system and say, 'What can we do?' I'm very quiet about it now. I spend a lot of time cheering for what I see, though, because I think what people are working on is really good."

The hospitals also have a role to play, and until recently have shirked their responsibility. It wasn't until June 1994, more than a year after the Commons sub-committee called for a national identification program, that the 1,200 hospitals of the Canadian Hospital Association drew up guidelines for a warning to blood users in the 1978–85 period to be checked.

What's the excuse? Did we really need the Commons report, a well-publicized fight for compensation for the victims of contaminated blood, and a major inquiry into the system to move hospitals into action? Had the battle for provincial assistance been lost and the governments held the line against the claimants, would testing ever have been done? If it takes that long to get such an urgent initiative going, with children maturing sexually and transfused patients infecting others, then the blood system surely is failing the Canadian people.

Some hospitals, notably the Hospital for Sick Children in Toronto, belatedly started their own programs to notify potential victims of tainted blood. Dr. Susan King, in charge of the program at Sick Kids, was asked during the Krever hearings about the implications of her discovery that 1 per cent of 1,700 child cardiac patients at the hospital were HIV-positive. Any big city in Canada, she said, could have similar rates of infection — Montreal, Vancouver, Ottawa, Edmonton — in cases of multiple transfusions of patients.

As the clamour over infection of hemophiliacs and the HIV-T group rose in late 1992 and early 1993, the hospital tried to track down children who had multiple transfusions in heart surgery before screening of blood began in late 1985. The testing started in April 1993, and a preliminary result in June reported six new cases had been found. When the early results were announced, King recalled the skepticism within the medical community that any new cases would be identified.

There was worse news to come. At the end of November, King reported that seventeen of the children had tested HIV-positive, a minimum of 1 per cent, because some families had not been tracked down. She also expected to find another seven among patients who had been treated for other problems than heart surgery. The grim toll among children treated at the hospital had now reached thirty HIV-positive cases. "This is certainly a higher incidence than many people expected," King remarked. She also said it would be reasonable to assume that adults would have a similar infection rate. Earlier, King had pointed out that half of a total of 17,000 children who had received blood transfusions at the hospital were now over sixteen and could be unknowingly infecting others through unprotected sex.

In September 1994, a group of Calgary researchers suggested a means of identifying HIV-infected blood donors that was stunning in its simplicity. Dr. John Gill of the University of Calgary, and Gwyneth Meyers and Amin Rajwani from the Southern Alberta AIDS clinic said doctors should ask all of their HIV-positive patients about their history of blood donations. With the patient's consent, doctors could then notify blood collection centres.

Since 1990, asking that straightforward question had become standard practice in southern Alberta, but the idea, the authors wrote in the *Canadian Medical Association Journal*, was "neglected in the published literature." Gill and colleagues had done a formal study of 478 HIV patients who paid routine visits to the clinic, and found that 112 could provide reliable data on their donations. Of those people,

32 were previously unknown to the Red Cross. Among the total of 545 units donated by the patients, 12 were a definite risk to the blood system, and another 57 were a possible risk. The study also indicated that although most of the HIV-positive donors voluntarily stopped giving blood, 12 were "either ill-informed or did not perceive themselves to be at risk." Only one person said he'd given blood simply to get an antibody test.

The director of the Red Cross National Testing Laboratory, Peter Gill (no relation to John Gill), said he liked the idea in an editorial in the same issue of the journal, and called for its universal adoption. Peter Gill also approved a proposal to give blood recipients all details of their transfusions when they leave the hospital, with an offer of follow-up tests six months to a year later. If that had been done in the 1980s, he noted, the burden on the health care system would have been much reduced.

Bob Pedersen, a former president of the Canadian Hemophilia Society, says he thinks the reluctance to track down people infected with HIV through blood was a litigation and public image issue. "They simply didn't want to go to court. Initially, I believe that in their arrogance they were confident that they could win lawsuits."

There are cost issues and political concerns surrounding notification. Health system authorities and doctors have talked about the massive costs involved in implementing a national testing program for blood-transfused people. And governments have been reluctant to talk about an embarrassing problem when they need to face the voters.

Blatant political manoeuvring was revealed at the Krever inquiry in June 1994, when Manitoba's chief medical officer said a call for blood-transfusion recipients to be tested was delayed in 1993 until five by-elections were held. The bulletin was held back for two months. The deputy minister of health for the province denied politics was the reason for the delay, but the allegation was investigated. During the campaign for those by-elections, health care cuts were a major issue. The government still lost all the seats.

The Commons sub-committee recommended in May 1993 that the federal health ministry "as a matter of urgency" take the lead in setting up a process to identify and notify HIV-positive blood-transfused persons. But the great Canadian excuse machine was working overtime. The tracing and notification of blood-transfused patients falls under provincial jurisdiction, said Joanne Ford, a Health and Welfare spokesperson, in late 1993. The Health Department had written the provinces in the summer of 1993 aiming to make the process more effective. There was no answer six months later, although some provinces had advised people who received transfusions in the critical period to be tested. But it's revealing that when the Health Department pounds the table over a tiny fee-for-service clinic in one province, the whole country hears it roar. On the issue of national notification of a group of unknown size infected by a fatal disease, its voice is, at best, a whisper.

The failure of the Red Cross, the hospitals, and governments to act in a timely way should not be tolerated. It is not good enough for these institutions to throw up their hands and say the process of lookback and notification of victims is terribly complicated. The issue is whether they even tried to find those who are infected. The plain fact is that they didn't try hard enough. In the full glare of adverse publicity, however, at least some have been shamed into action.

The numbers potentially at risk are stunning in their magnitude. It's estimated that 600,000 residents of Ontario and 400,000 in Quebec received blood transfusions in that critical period between 1978 and 1985. Why did that June 1994 announcement to test those who had received transfusions not come a year earlier, at least?

Governments, those purported guardians of public safety, cannot wash their hands of this scandal. Politicians fondly believed responsibility lay elsewhere. But government must protect its citizens. Instead, the politicians and bureaucrats preferred to pass the buck. The notification fiasco is today's reminder of what went wrong with the system in the 1980s. These vestiges indicate reform is needed. While the faces in charge may change, the issues remain almost identical.

Chapter 11

DREAM ROBBERS

"I'm here to tell you about the dream robbers. And the thief of our dreams is not AIDS. AIDS is only a symptom. It is not the disease itself; it is the structures within our society that caused AIDS to be spread among the marginalized. Those structures silence us. When we share our pain, when we tell our stories, we are treated with either scorn or pity."

LORRAINE CALDERWOOD-PARSONS, IN A LECTURE, 1994

It was a sunny Saturday in the spring of 1986. The date is hard to remember, but the news is impossible to forget.

David, our fifteen-year-old son, sat on the couch in our family room. He spoke quietly and that made the horror of what he was telling us all the more stark.

David had gone to the hemophilia clinic at the Ottawa General Hospital for what was ostensibly a routine six-month check-up. He had scanned down the nurse's chart and had seen "HIV-positive." That was good, right? Positive had to be good!

The nurse took him aside and broke the news to him — a young teenager, alone, unexpectedly crushed under the burden of finding out that he had tested positive for the virus that causes AIDS.

His mother and I hadn't thought anything of it when he left for his check-up that Saturday morning. David was old enough now to attend clinic on his own. He was at an age, indeed, when youth resents hovering parents.

Hemophilia meant nothing to me in 1969. As a history buff, I was vaguely aware of some connection of the "bleeder's disease" to the royal families of Europe. It wasn't until I met my future wife,

Lorraine Calderwood, in Newfoundland that it ever occurred to me that it would play an enormous role in my life.

Lorraine had experience with its dreadful consequences. Her father, Roy, had died from a hemorrhage when she was five, and her widowed mother struggled in a small northern British Columbia town to build a career while raising five fun-loving and strong-willed daughters. Lorraine's eldest sister has a young son who almost died from a bleed when he was a toddler. When she went off to Carleton University in Ottawa to study journalism, Lorraine chose to write on hemophilia as her undergraduate thesis.

As our romance blossomed, we talked occasionally about what hemophilia would mean to us if we were to start a family. There was a fifty-fifty chance a son would be a hemophiliac and the same risk that daughters would be carriers of the hemophilic gene. She spoke about the excruciating pain a hemophiliac could suffer as blood seeped into the joints, pushing them apart. But there was hope. Only a few years before, there had been the discovery of cryoprecipitate, the fraction of plasma that carried an enriched quantity of the missing blood-clotting agent, Factor VIII.

Perhaps it was the bravado of a young man, but the chance of having this genetic disease in my family was not about to scare me away from this interesting young woman. Besides, there was hope! Life would be better for families with hemophilia. And so we married in December 1969 in her hometown of Smithers, British Columbia.

In the summer of 1970, Lorraine found she was pregnant. A doctor, knowing of her family background, offered an abortion. Horrified, Lorraine declined. This was a child that would be wanted and loved.

When friends asked if we wanted a boy or a girl, Lorraine said she just wanted the baby to be healthy. In retrospect, that comment went over my head. I certainly agreed, but always leaned towards a girl. My excuse was that I had always wanted a sister, and a daughter would be like the female sibling I never had. Privately, although the rationalizations of youth fade away with age, I'm sure I feared for the consequences if it might be a male child.

I was with Lorraine in the Ottawa delivery room when our first baby was born. As the infant's head emerged into the wide world, the doctor first exclaimed, "It's a girl!" I don't know if he was teasing or whether it was the baby's good looks that led him to that erroneous conclusion. Whatever, my heart jumped with joy. But the rest of the newcomer's body brought a reversal of opinion. "No, it's a boy!" I can't say that I was any less happy.

Our son, David Roy, was born in April 1971.

After our David was born, the doctor assured us that he was perfectly healthy. It was difficult to test the blood of infants for levels of clotting factor, we were told, but there was nothing to worry about. We were put at ease and forgot about the possibility he might be a hemophiliac.

Several months after David was born, however, I received a frantic call at work from Lorraine. There was something terribly wrong. The baby had been screaming all afternoon, one leg drawn up in pain. David was taken to the hospital where he was examined and blood samples taken.

The news was not long in coming. David was a severe Factor VIII hemophiliac. It would mean long nights spent in hospitals, a lifelong disease with no cure in sight, needles, pressure bandages, ice packs, restricted activities. Dr. Marc Robinson told us, however, about the advances in treatment. He encouraged us to try to live life as normally as possible, and said that there was a society for hemophiliacs where we could get more information. That night was long, restless, and tearful.

As David grew, he turned out to be an adventuresome and inquisitive child. This is true of many hemophiliacs. It's as if they are challenging life, daring it to test them to the fullest. Naturally, this also meant frequent visits to the hospital — at first the old Ottawa General just off Sussex Drive — to treat hemorrhages in knees, ankles, elbows, and muscles. A tumble down the stairs, life-threatening for any child, became for us a nightmarish threat. We spent hour after hour in the emergency room of that institution, before being given word that it was okay to take him home and just to watch for symptoms of internal bleeding.

It was hard to leave him behind on overnight stays, which occurred once every couple of months. There was nowhere in the crowded, aging building for parents to stay. David would bellow when we left. He had a loud, distinctive voice that we could pick out well down the hallway. Often, the nurses would put up white padding all around David's cot. We don't know whether that was because they were afraid that, as a hemophiliac, he would bruise his head on the bars, or whether they wanted to block his view of us leaving for home. But it was a sterile environment and Lorraine started taping pictures to the padding to give him something to look at.

The hospital visits were hard to bear and not only for David's sake. It was overwhelming sometimes to see young children with bald heads suffering from leukemia and the hydrocephalic kids confined to their beds. At times like that we were almost thankful our child "only" had hemophilia. But the visits took a toll on Lorraine and me. Sometimes, weary of the long waits in the middle of the night with a child in pain and fed up dealing with the ignorance of emergency room doctors, we would quarrel over whose turn it was to go to the hospital. Often, doctors and nurses would have trouble inserting needles in David's small veins for the infusion of blood-coagulating cryoprecipitate. Several of them would gather around the young toddler and poke him up to five or six times before being successful. On several occasions, as David howled in pain, they would order us to leave the room. Rather than subject him to that treatment, we would lie down beside David at home to comfort him, pack his knee or ankle with ice, and hope the bleeding would stop. It seldom worked.

No wonder that when David played "doctor," he would take his teddy bear or another stuffed animal and pile all his other toys on top of it. That was his notion of what medical treatment meant.

The reactions of friends and others we encountered were mixed. Some parents at a day care centre that David attended didn't want their children to play with him. Perhaps they were afraid their child would hurt him; some may even have feared that hemophilia was contagious. But occasionally old myths about the bleeding disease surfaced: You must have royal blood, or equally preposterous, there must be inbreeding in your family to have a hemophiliac child. The hardest reactions to contend with were the stares you got in public whenever David had a nasty-looking bruise on his face or arms. Every parent of a severe hemophiliac child knows those looks.

In March 1976, David fell and hit his head in the school yard where he attended junior kindergarten. He was sent home on the school bus vomiting and suffering from a severe headache. Lorraine took him to Ottawa's Children's Hospital of Eastern Ontario, where he was kept in overnight for observation, given cryoprecipitate, and discharged the next morning. She was given a card listing symptoms that, if observed, should prompt a return to hospital.

Lorraine returned several times to the hospital with David over the next week, concerned that his increasing malaise, headaches, and the tingling sensation in his feet were signs of internal bleeding. The hematologists dismissed her fears. On one occasion, a doctor asked David if he had been jumping up and down that day. When David said yes, the doctor concluded that was the cause of the tingling in the feet and sent him packing. A week later, David ate a single hot dog for supper — this in itself was unusual, as he loved hot dogs and usually would put away three. He fell asleep immediately after supper and awoke vomiting. The next day, when Lorraine was visiting her own doctor, he started screaming and claiming he couldn't walk. At home, he lapsed into unconsciousness.

David was rushed to hospital, but the doctors still seemed reluctant to consider the possibility of bleeding from the previous head injury. Dr. Brian Luke, the chief hematologist, suggested it was the flu, food poisoning, or meningitis that was causing David's illness. Luke didn't order a CAT scan for David until a brother-in-law, also a doctor, called from Edmonton to complain. The scan identified two blood clots on his brain. When medication proved ineffective, it was decided surgery — a craniotomy — was necessary. To our knowledge, David was the first Canadian severe hemophiliac to survive that kind of operation, thanks to the blood-clotting agents. But the accident left him with learning and motor-skill disabilities. He had to learn to walk again, and he switched from being right-handed to left-handed at a time when most children were just learning the skills of printing and drawing.

Later, we complained to the Ontario College of Physicians and Surgeons about the medical treatment. They brushed off the complaint, but we took it a step further to the Ontario Health Disciplines Board. The board sent the scenario, with all identifying references deleted, to a hemophilia specialist who decided the doctors should have assumed an intracranial hemorrhage "until proven otherwise." The board called for the doctors involved to be admonished for their sloppy treatment. This experience suggested to us that in many cases, parents of children with chronic disease have a better sense of what can go wrong than the so-called experts.

We were stunned at how the Hemophilia Society reacted. Someone in the media who knew us identified David as the child in the Health Disciplines Board decision and an in-depth story on the affair appeared two days running in the *Ottawa Citizen*. Other media picked it up as well. Then we were shocked to hear the local chairman of the Society — who has since died of AIDS — defending the doctors on CBC radio by saying, "They did all they could." The case was brought to the Ontario CHS board, but they decided to do nothing. They did not want to get involved in a "political" issue. We were also upset when Luke was named to the CHS medical and scientific advisory committee. Frankly, we were disgusted at the conservatism of the society and wanted nothing to do with it for several years.

But raising a stink has other consequences. We did not want to deal again with those doctors whose "low index of suspicion"— to put it politely — had almost killed our son, so we asked to return to the Ottawa General for his hemophilia treatment. This was agreeable to the staff there for a while. But then heat was put on the doctors at the General. Children in Ottawa must be treated at the Children's Hospital, they were told. David had no choice. You will do what you can to protect your kids, so we decided to pack our bags and move someplace where we had heard there was better treatment. In late 1978 we decided to move to Vancouver, and fortunately our employers were open to moving us.

This was a good choice. David's lack of coordination meant he had frequent hemorrhages in his legs. In Vancouver, not only was there a full-fledged hemophilia program, but David was put on prophylactic doses of clotting agent and given an intensive exercise program. After about a year, his knees were almost back to normal.

When we first moved to Vancouver in December 1978, the standard treatment for hemophilia was still cryoprecipitate, which had to be packed in dry ice for short trips and required a complicated apparatus to administer. Soon, we were to learn of the miracle of dried, powdered clotting factors that allowed us to travel. We took an extended trip one summer to California and even into Tijuana, Mexico, safe in the knowledge that if David had a problem we had the concentrate with us. I especially remember pulling over in the stifling-hot Mojave Desert to give him an injection, amazed at what a liberating product it was.

While in British Columbia, I became involved in the Canadian Hemophilia Society again. A member of the B.C. board knew I was a reporter and persuaded me to play a role in the media relations plan for the Society's national convention in Vancouver. That's where I met Bill Rudd, then the provincial president but soon to go on to become the national leader of the CHS. He later played a significant role in the acquisition of heat-treated blood products. Unfortunately, Bill has since died. Bill Rudd encouraged me to become B.C. president, and I held that role in 1980 and 1981 until I was transferred by my employer to Toronto.

It was after the move to Toronto that I first heard of the possibility that hemophiliacs were among the groups vulnerable to the mysterious disease known as AIDS. A twenty-nine-year-old B.C. hemophiliac was one of the first in Canada to be infected and die from AIDS complications in March 1983, according to Federal Centre for AIDS statistics, but that didn't become common knowledge until a year later when an inquest was held into his death. Even today, authorities in the blood system largely ignore that young man's existence and his untimely fate. With a nudge and a wink, they suggest there were "other factors" involved. All we know for sure is that he was a hemophiliac.

Certainly, at that time few hemophiliacs seemed to be concerned. Some, indeed, attacked the media for linking blood with AIDS. A common refrain was that there was a risk of AIDS through blood contamination but it was exceptionally rare. The infamous "one-in-a-million" line about the chance of infection, which had first found root in the United States, was being repeated in Canada.

Early in 1983, our brother-in-law who had intervened to help save David in 1976 told us to avoid Factor VIII concentrates produced from blood of American origin. This was not an off-the-cuff remark. He is a pediatrician with two hemophiliac sons. The reaction of one staff member at the Hospital for Sick Children's blood bank when I made the request for "Canadian only" was interesting, however. He sniggered and gave me a scornful look that suggested I was some kind of ignorant troublemaker.

I found out many years later that others had reached the same conclusion and by insisting on Canadian-source product or cryoprecipitate managed to avoid HIV. It's startling to think that so many blood experts failed to grasp that simple idea and continued to defend the integrity of the blood system.

But hemophiliacs and their parents are used to this kind of shoddy treatment by those in authority. Ask them. They'll all have tales to tell of rotten treatment or sneering condescension at even top-of-the-line hospitals. The best doctors are those who realize that people used to coping with lifelong disease very likely know more about the condition than they do.

Ask mothers who take their young hemophiliac children to emergency rooms for treatment of bleeds if the words "mother hysterical" have appeared on charts because they demanded quick treatment. What many interns can't seem to grasp is that the faster you treat hemophiliacs — and a doctor doesn't have to do it personally, nurses will do — the faster you get them out of the waiting-room or off the examination table they occupy. Delay treatment, and the pain and damage mount and more costly care is required.

There's no wonder that a recent survey of hemophiliacs ranked "Receiving emergency treatment from unknowledgeable professionals" as one of their biggest fears. And 60 per cent of the respondents said that situation had happened to them.

Usually the smugness on the part of authorities, medical or non-medical, is merely insulting or results in a hour or two delay in proper treatment. Sometimes it can mean more pain and agony for the sufferers of the disease. Occasionally, it can have fatal consequences, as in the case of those who could not accept — even when the evidence was clear — that HIV infection would mean death for those who received tainted blood products.

One reason the news of David's HIV-positive test came as such a shock was that in December 1985 we had been told that David had a test at the Hospital for Sick Children in Toronto showing he was HIV-negative. I had left that session rejoicing that he was safe from the fatal disease, even though the doctor cautioned that it was still not certain what a positive or a negative test meant. I had told Lorraine of the results — her initial view when we gave consent for the test had been that she didn't want to know the results. But since the Toronto test was good news, why hold it back?

So, instead of going to the clinic, where we could have offered our son support that terrible Saturday, we stayed at home. I was spray-painting some furniture in the garage and Lorraine was working in the kitchen.

My initial reaction was disbelief. The positive test must be a mistake, I said. We'll ask for a retest. After all, the new heat-treated products had been distributed exclusively, we were told, for a year now, long before David's previous negative test. A retest was done, but the news was the same. David was positive. Still, we could not reconcile ourselves to the possibility that this could be fatal. It seemed so unfair for someone who had dealt with disabilities all his short life to be hit again.

Our astonishment was compounded on December 29, 1994 — the date of our twenty-fifth wedding anniversary — when we received a letter by courier from the Hospital for Sick Children. For over two years I had been requesting information to try to reconcile apparent gaps in David's tests. From what we had been told, we had long believed David was a late infection, likely contaminated after the introduction of heat-treated products. In March 1994 we were sent a sixteen-page compilation of records by Sick Kids, which we were told included "all the test results." But something didn't add up. There didn't seem to be any specific test for HIV in the package. We wrote letters and made phone calls trying to find out more. We were unaware that in the fall of 1994, the Canadian Hemophilia Society had also asked the hospital to divulge to patients any HIV test results that were not included in patient files.

The December 1994 letter informed us for the first time of the results of another serum sample taken at Sick Kids in June 1985, coded, and tested anonymously for HIV by Dr. Michael O'Shaughnessy at Ottawa's Laboratory Centre for Disease Control (LCDC). We do not recall ever having specifically consented to that test, although we did receive a form letter in September 1985 thanking us for "allowing David to participate in our Immune Surveillance Study of hemophiliacs." The 1985 letter mentioned that one test to be performed was "a measurement of antibody to a specific virus (HTLV-III) that is thought to be the cause of AIDS." It continued: "Obviously, if we find abnormal results or have concerns about your son's health, we will be discussing these issues directly with you (unless you specifically instruct us not to do so)." We were never told of the abnormal results until December 1994.

"The first sample from June 24, 1985, was reported positive for antibodies to HIV," Dr. Victor Blanchette wrote. "A further serum sample dated December 16, 1985, tested negative for antibodies. The third sample from June 6, 1986, was reported positive." All had been tested at the LCDC. Blanchette said that several years after the June 1985 sample was submitted, it was retested by O'Shaughnessy and confirmed positive through the ELISA and Western Blot tests. "With the advantage of this information, it is my opinion that David was HIV-infected at a time prior to June 1985," the letter says.

We will always wonder when he was infected. One of the groups given priority to receive heat-treated products under the recommendations from the Hemophilia Society's medical advisors in the spring of 1985 was previously treated hemophiliacs known to be seronegative. Why wasn't David tested before May 1985 — when the safe products were first on hand at Red Cross centres — to determine if he fit into that group? If the heat-treated products had been distributed earlier, could he have escaped contamination? Many people still lack answers to these crucial questions.

"It was difficult going to school after that," David says today. "It was like I didn't know what to think about it. I couldn't really talk to anybody about it back then. It would have caused a lot of fear in the school, having a classmate who was HIV-positive and all that stuff. So I just stayed quiet about it. I did tell one friend, and he went around and told other people. That kind of hurt. I forgive him for that now, but I was pissed off that he did that."

The impact of finding out that you, or someone close, has an infection that can lead to AIDS affects people differently. Like David, Lorraine and I submerged it. We did not discuss what this would mean to David or how it would affect our own lives. The only time I thought about it much over the next two years was once when I accidentally poked myself with one of David's needles. I asked for a test; it came back negative.

Lorraine and I seldom discussed the almost certain possibility that David would get AIDS. It was almost as though we believed the disease would disappear if we never broached the subject. We did not tell our friends or David's two younger sisters. If anyone asked about it, we looked them straight in the eye and told a barefaced lie. Was that the appropriate response? Who can say? When we hear of the families whose homes were spray-painted with graffiti or attacked, who were verbally abused, whose kids were barred from schools and who lost their jobs, it may well have been. Today, with the Krever inquiry into the blood supply and the persistent news coverage of blood-transfused AIDS, the climate for talking about the disease is generally better. David is selective about who he tells. "Why put something stressful on a person when there's no reason to?" he asks.

But back then, David, too, put it out of his mind, although he remembers coming home from high school two years after that fateful Saturday and saying to himself, Hey, I guess I'm not going to die. At the time, it was widely believed if one didn't die within two years, there was a chance of survival.

After that, David began drinking heavily and using drugs. Still, he kept a generally even keel in his relationships outside the home. Teachers found him polite and cooperative, as did medical professionals. He worked hard to complete Grade 12 — much of that year was spent in a hospital bed. But his outlet for the rage inside was at home. He would boil over with anger at his parents, and occasionally he would leave the house for a few days, or we would order him out. He often wandered the streets, playing his guitar on corners for a few dollars. Street life was rough. Several times David was beaten up and he was robbed — both of the few dollars he had earned and of his precious guitar. Early one Saturday morning I was called to pick up a surly, disruptive patient from hospital. I almost didn't recognize his battered face.

Meanwhile, there was other upsetting news to absorb in the late 1980s. There are four hemophiliacs in the extended family. Three of them, including David, were found to be HIV-positive.

None of us dealt with the issue well. I was asked in 1988 to help develop a media relations strategy for the Canadian Hemophilia Society's request to the federal government for compensation. It was a tricky task, particularly because the Society wanted its message to get across without exposing the individual human element that makes such appeals effective. I participated with greater reluctance than I would today, I confess. Lorraine went to some women's support meetings, and both of us became more involved with the Society again. David's participation was limited to youth activities, including one trip to Vancouver, which for him and some others who were HIV-infected, turned into a drinking spree.

We had also kept the secret from David's sisters, Jennifer and Jill, which was a mistake. When Jenny, then a troubled sixteen-year-old, was finally told, she moved out of our home; she now lives in British Columbia. It wasn't until Christmas 1994, when Jenny visited with her infant daughter — our first grandchild — that there was a full reconciliation. Over those years, however, Jenny had seen David when he visited her, and she clearly never stopped loving her brother.

As for Jill, we got up the nerve to break the news to her after attending a couples retreat put on by the Canadian Hemophilia Society in Orillia in 1992. She's now quite active in the Society, made a moving pitch for safer blood products before the Canadian Blood Agency when she was fifteen, and also participates in local AIDS activities.

When David received his first year of federal compensation money, it fuelled his self-destructive binge. In a drunken stupor, he handed out cash to any hanger-on who asked. In one wild day and night in Calgary, he gave a thousand dollars to street people and a varied assortment of barflies. This $30,000, wrung from the government through the hard work of hemophiliacs and supporters, was being squandered when it might be needed later for medicines and nursing care.

David travelled twice to Europe, the first time on money he earned from a part-time job. On the first occasion, he dwelt in decadence until his money ran out and then lived in barefoot poverty. If the Belgian police hadn't insisted that this scruffy, shoeless, ill-clad, syringe-carrying vision of John the Baptist get on board a plane, no self-respecting airline would have carried him back to Canada.

David also went twice to Nicaragua, where he found a sense of mission with people who, like him, were hurting. Nicaragua may indeed have been a turning point. David first went with me in 1988 as part of a group from Holy Cross Catholic Church in Ottawa, which has a sister parish just outside Managua. Although David barely spoke a word of Spanish, somehow he struck a chord with the young people in one of the poorest barrios there. By and large, these were people living in makeshift wood and black plastic houses, driven to the capital by the contra war raging in the rural areas. David spent a lot of time with them and saw more of their day-to-day life than we adults did. He got to know Amalia, a young woman who has since become a nurse. At the time, she was held back by the brace she had to wear on a leg affected by polio. She wrote him letters, and has become a close friend.

He says his three visits to Nicaragua raised his morale. There's a strong sense of community in the barrios, stronger than in North America where people seem absorbed by the fight to get ahead. "People know how to work together and value community. Those are more important to them than having lots of money."

Since then, he has raised $1,000 for a school in Managua, collected and sent to Central America surplus wheelchairs and crutches from Ottawa hospitals, and become a sponsor for a young boy in Colombia.

David has also quit drinking and using drugs. Late one Saturday night he came home and announced he wasn't going to drink or use drugs anymore. I gave him a hug, not quite believing it. But he has stuck to that promise.

David's great love in high school was his theatre class. He had a facility for fitting into a role, really getting inside the role he was playing. His teachers recognized this talent, and one of them still uses a character that he created in her class.

In 1990, the year David graduated from Grade 12, the high school play was *Les Misérables*. David had a small part as a constable, but he played the role with such intensity and power that they expanded the part. I remember that the administrator of Ottawa's Great Canadian Theatre Company attended the play the same night we were there. You can imagine the pride when she said that when David was on stage, she could not take her eyes away from him.

During the second-to-last performance, David felt something was wrong with his ankle. He played the first half but was unable to continue after the intermission. We brought some Factor VIII for him, which seemed to alleviate the problem for a time. Still, he was unable to perform the next day.

Over the next four or five days, we continued to treat David's bad ankle as a hemorrhage. He was in extreme and increasing pain over that time; the concentrate just didn't seem to be working. We had bought David a reclining chair a few years before. On nights when he had hemorrhages in his legs, it was far more comfortable for him to sleep in a sitting position than lying in a bed. This time nothing seemed to work. He was in utter agony and his ankle kept swelling up. He had to be helped to the bathroom, and a couple of nights one of us stayed up and slept on the couch while David rested fitfully on the chair.

Finally, we took him to hospital. One of the doctors decided that to relieve the pressure from what was thought to be the leaking blood, he would aspirate fluid through a needle from the ankle joint. But when the fluid was drawn, there was no blood. He didn't have a hemorrhage at all! A decision was made to operate and clean the septic ankle out. It took six weeks before David was out of the hospital, and for a long time after that he had to walk with a cane.

David has since been told by a doctor that the infection was likely related to his HIV status. You learn a lot from talking to other people. Septic infections in joints seem to be a common occurrence among HIV-positive hemophiliacs, showing up long before opportunistic infections. "It's weird," David says, "because back then I was pretty healthy, and that's how suddenly this virus can affect your life."

Perhaps as parents we over-react. But with that incident, we began to worry about illnesses that to anyone else might seem routine. A cough, a sore throat, a headache — all became potential threats. Some opportunistic infections are scarcely known to the experts, let alone the average doctor or nurse. Who knows where they might lead? With HIV-AIDS, there are so many ways health can be put at risk.

From a parent's viewpoint, we have trouble reconciling his HIV status with his desire to spend time in Central America. With a compromised immune system, he has been warned, trips to Third World countries could put him at risk of fatal infection, or sap his strength. But if AIDS is fatal, why shouldn't he enjoy his life and engage in activities in which he feels he is contributing. It's truly a dilemma. We want him to be happy in the time he has, but fear for the future.

For hemophiliacs and other blood-transfused people living with HIV and AIDS, it is galling to think there are people out there who could have stopped this tragedy but who failed in their duty to protect the public. Within the same day in early March 1994, David found his T-cell count had dropped sharply from a previous test and also was told the Factor VIII lot that infected him might have been identified.

As it turns out, he may never know the truth about that lot number. David did receive concentrate from at least two lots of Cutter Factor VIII — one commercially produced and numbered 50P020 — that had been distributed by the Red Cross in August 1985 and had not been screened for the virus. We never received a recall notice for that product, even though one was sent out in 1987. The Red Cross told us by letter that later investigations of the lot by Health Canada found the recalled Cutter products were not implicated in any cases of HIV transmission. They also said no samples of the lot remain, so it may never be proven unless something comes to light in the future. We know, too, that David used nearly twenty other vials from the sixty-seven Armour and Cutter lots that were recalled in late 1987 after seven hemophiliacs were infected in Western Canada. These unscreened although heat-treated products were distributed to him as late as July 1987 by the Ottawa General Hospital. Apparently, he did not receive any of the three lots specifically implicated, but hemophiliacs have been told half-truths or had information withheld from them so often that, for us, doubt will never be fully dispelled.

That combination of news enraged him. "It was scary when I found out my count was constantly dropping. I felt very angry that day. I felt like putting bombs at the Red Cross and blowing the place up. I try to stay hopeful, and go on with life. But I realize I could die of AIDS. I don't want to die, because I'm too young, and I also think about the other people who died and who are suffering because of negligence in the Red Cross.

"You see people being devalued for selfish reasons or for money, or whatever, by government and the Red Cross. It's like they're not concerned. They don't think these are real people. How would you feel — would you like to be dying of AIDS? What if your wife or your child or your brother got AIDS? They thought about how they could spend the least money. How they could make it easier for themselves. They were completely corrupt. And then they didn't recall the factors even after they started screening the blood supplies. They just kept giving it out, because it was easier and: 'Oh, well, some people might get infected, but not very many.' This was something really evil, or at least not very morally intact.

"I wouldn't put bombs at the Red Cross, but things like that come to the imagination. And why not? People are killed for less, that's for sure. And acts of terrorism are committed for less."

David went to the YMCA and worked off his anger. "I felt better afterwards. That was a hard workout."

David is philosophical about his lot today, probably more so than his parents. He prefers to use his energy constructively, taking courses, learning Spanish, doing volunteer work. "It's a drag to be angry all the time," he says.

"I prefer to focus on a positive lifestyle. It's not so much that I want to be unconcerned about HIV, but I don't want to be preoccupied by it. I want to be concerned enough about it that I will keep it in mind and use it in a positive sense. Keep going and taking risks and staying in shape."

Occasionally, the negative side intrudes and he admits to being scared. "Sometimes I think, What's the point of life? I don't think of it in a suicidal or sad way. I'm not one of those types that go off and say, Woe is me!"

Parents, spouses, children, siblings, and friends often feel the anger even more than those who are HIV-infected. There's a sense of injustice, that unpunished and unrepentant criminals are on the loose, some still running the system. Lawyers have said it is frequently the relatives who have wanted to pursue court action to the bitter end, even if the chances of victory are slight. Usually, the ill don't have the energy to continue. Emotions spin from fury to bottomless anguish to abject helplessness to a sense of betrayal to sickening fear that the next cough or bout of diarrhea could be the beginning of the end.

We have felt all of those sentiments and more in our family. We have been driven to track down the blood lot that damaged our son through the endless bureaucracy, even though he has accepted the government compensation and there is no thought of litigation. When the subject of HIV and hemophilia arose in conversation with friends and workmates, we have felt guilt as we brazenly lied to them — either because the time to tell was not right or we were afraid of the reaction. We have witnessed the pain our son has felt through discrimination at the hands of a local doctor while he was attending college in Sault Ste. Marie, and the discrimination suffered by a nephew at a British Columbia school. We have learned a friend with whom David was sharing an apartment told him to leave when he found out David was HIV-positive. We have nagged David endlessly to take pills that make him nauseated until finally he put his foot down and told us where to go. We have waited apprehensively on a New Year's Eve for word of that treasured nephew, Mischa, who was close to death but thankfully recovered. We have seen the pain in a daughter's eyes when we finally summoned the courage to tell her that her only brother was inflicted with a preventable, fatal disease. And we have wept angry tears, and leaned on the courage of others, when we have heard the stories of those in our broadening community who have passed away.

Pat O'Connor, a man of great personal courage, summed it up. He realized when he told his parents that he was infected that any parent's biggest fear is losing one of their children. It's true. It happens often in life, of course, but that doesn't make it any easier to bear when it's your own child.

Chapter 12

SEARCH FOR JUSTICE

*"We'd better get going on behalf of our people, because
some of them are going to die."*

ED KUBIN, 1987

Ed Kubin has been credited by some with starting the ball rolling in
the fight for compensation for the victims of bad blood.

In the aftermath of the blood contamination disaster, the Canadian Hemophilia Society, under president Bob Pedersen of Hamilton,
Ontario, set up a task force to decide what programs were needed to
help hemophiliacs and their families. Kubin, a Manitoba hemophiliac who had been national secretary in 1985, was on the task force.

Bob O'Neill, former national program director for the Canadian
Hemophilia Society, recalls a meeting in 1987 when Kubin, never one
to mince words, said aloud what some others had been thinking: "I
blame those bastards in Ottawa." A federal Health Department
employee, attending the meeting, was horrified and reported to her
superiors.

O'Neill was called after that by a federal official who told him
that if hemophiliacs wanted help, Kubin would have to be removed
from the task force. "We can't put up with people who threaten violence against the government," O'Neill recalls him saying. "I said I
was a bit nervous about Ed myself, but now I've made up my mind.
I didn't want somebody in government saying who can be on our
committee. So I said, 'Ed is on.'"

Pedersen, too, remembers Kubin's intervention when there was a discussion of getting the doctors and clinics prepared for the expected onslaught of ill hemophiliacs. Kubin is "a very strong-spoken gentleman" not averse to using the odd profanity, Pedersen says.

"To hell with the medical community," Pedersen remembers Kubin saying. "Let's take care of our own. There's compensation going to happen worldwide, in civilized countries anyway; we'd better get going on behalf of our people, because some of them are going to die. They're not going to be around to have any bloody benefits from their physicians."

"It was such a well-spoken and hard-assed position that I for one took it up, as did a couple of other people who said we have to change our attitude and move into compensation as the major AIDS care issue," Pedersen says. "The central motivating factor was Mr. Ed Kubin, redirecting the entire organization with a couple of key sentences."

Meanwhile, David Page of Quebec, then the CHS program director, was invited to lunch one day by Chris Tsoukas, the Montreal immunologist who had participated in a study on the immune status of several severe hemophiliacs. Tsoukas's father had died young, and Chris had to struggle for years to reach his ambition of becoming a doctor. "Many kids are going to be losing their fathers," Tsoukas told Page. "The Society must do something so they won't have to go through what I went through." The doctor played a large role in the coming campaign. Page says the eminent immunologist increased CHS credibility with the federal Health Department.

About the same time, Sudbury hemophiliac Bob Gibson had started talking about approaching the provincial government for compensation. So in May 1987, the CHS executive adopted financial relief for families affected by HIV as its prime "social rights" objective, and the fight for compensation was on.

The Society began compiling the necessary background and documentation to fight its case. Sub-committees were established to do archival research to try to predict the numbers of people infected and how much it would take to care for them for the remainder of their lives. They studied the linkages among the Red Cross, the Bureau of Biologics, the federal Health Department, and the Canadian Blood Committee. A lobbying group and a strategic planning committee were also set up. Gibson, who was HIV-infected, was chosen chairman of the campaign until he became too ill to continue and was replaced by Page, later a national CHS president.

An actuarial analysis was prepared by the Winnipeg firm Eckler Partners Limited, and a legal opinion sought from Heenan Blaikie, the Montreal law firm of former prime minister Pierre Trudeau. The archival search was a monumental task undertaken by Gibson and Stephen Christmas, who have both since died. It traced the origins of the blood system and sought to determine how it failed when confronted by the threat of contaminated blood. A hemophilia population survey was conducted, affected members were asked to write letters, and lobbying efforts began with government and opposition members of Parliament. Meanwhile, disability income and survivor benefits were established as the main targets. At that time, it was expected that most of those infected would only live a couple of years longer.

A year after the process had begun, much of the preparatory work was complete. A medical report noted the extent of immune deficiency and HIV infection among hemophiliacs. Heenan Blaikie's preliminary opinion was that the failure of the Red Cross to adequately advise holders of the defective concentrates subject to recall "would appear to create liability" based on an earlier Supreme Court ruling that there is a continuing duty to warn consumers of danger after distribution. The firm also warned, however, that more research would be required to look at the implications for dispensing institutions such as hospitals and clinics. Many hemophiliacs were of the opinion, in any case, that pursuit through the courts would only add to stress felt by those who were ill and many victims could not afford the expense. A study argued that hemophiliacs, generally excluded from obtaining insurance because of their condition, were already under financial stress from their HIV infection. Existing social services were not enough to cover the extra costs of diet, clothing, and special care needed by those suffering from the effects of the virus.

After receiving some heat from the gay community following an early brochure, the CHS had changed the name of its campaign to "catastrophe relief" from "compensation." The offending leaflet had called for assistance to the "victims" of HIV, apparently restricting this phrase to those contaminated through blood. Gay leaders said everybody was a victim, recalls Elaine Woloschuk, a Windsor, Ontario, mother of a hemophiliac and teacher who replaced Pedersen as national CHS president. "They said nobody should be singled out as a special victim, and if there was any compensation, they should all be entitled to compensation. We drew a parallel between a natural disaster and a medical disaster, where nobody was truly at fault. We didn't want to lay the blame at anybody's feet but we really wanted to highlight the issue, and look to the government for compassion in financial support, just the way others do who experience natural disaster such as earthquake, fire, hurricane, and drought that wipes out farmers' crops."

A later brochure said "compensation" implied restitution for some wrong and that until legal questions were clarified, it could not be certain that anyone was legally to blame. "That the hemophilia community has suffered a catastrophe is beyond all doubt. That this catastrophe occurred for reasons out of our control is also obvious. And it is clear that the affected individuals and their families need relief."

One of Pedersen's final acts as CHS president had been to inform Jake Epp, then health minister in Brian Mulroney's government, that the Society would be making a request for catastrophe relief. Over the summer of 1988, the assorted studies supporting the assistance proposal were completed and a summary document prepared. Fortuitously, Britain had announced a compensation package for its 1,200 infected hemophiliacs and the Royal Society of Canada had put out a special report on AIDS in Canada that recommended persons infected with HIV through blood transfusions or blood products be compensated. (One of the contributors to that report was Judge Horace Krever, later to head the national inquiry into the blood system.)

The summary, prepared by Bob O'Neill, pointed out that of 1,000 infected hemophiliacs, 840 had little or no life insurance, 620 had no group insurance, 504 were having difficulty at work or at school, and 420 already had increased medical costs. By 1993, it predicted, half of the infected would be dead and four-fifths of the rest would be severely ill. The actuarial study put the total cost of the CHS proposal, including disability, survivors' benefits, a lump-sum payment, and other items, at between $330 and $400 million.

Elaine Woloschuk, described by Pedersen as one of the most politically astute players in the CHS, led the delegation from the society into the meeting with Epp on August 15, 1988. The "world's best teacher," according to some of her students, was quiet, cool, and confident. But Epp seemed skeptical. He suggested the Society would have to show it had public support behind it.

"I think he was trying to make a connection between HIV and hemophilia and the gay community," says Woloschuk, who remembers him asking how many infected hemophiliacs might be gay.

"I assume that the same proportion of people within the hemophilia community as among the broader community," she replied. "If 10 or 15 per cent of the broader population is gay, I would imagine that 10 to 15 per cent of the hemophilia community would be gay. What's your reason for asking?"

"Well, is it all those people who are infected?" Epp asked.

"I wouldn't begin to answer that question," Woloschuk replied. "Our claim was that people were infected because of the blood product and not because of their association with a particular lifestyle or sexual orientation. He didn't like that answer."

The dealings with Epp were to be short-lived. At the end of September, a federal election was called and when Mulroney's Conservatives came back, Epp was shuffled off to another ministry. The last question in the Commons before the election call came was from Liberal Sheila Copps to Epp, probing his response to the CHS appeal. He gave a non-committal answer.

The Catastrophe Relief Committee was not about to let a little thing like a federal election stop the momentum. Supporters were encouraged to question candidates on whether they backed compensation for hemophiliacs. Letters were written, and the society requested donors to send in tear-off cards to the government. Woloschuk says between 20,000 and 30,000 cards were sent.

"There was still a lot of fear of discrimination," she says. At that point, the national CHS started to shift its strategy and began linking hemophilia and AIDS. Until then, the public position had been that the two were not related. "But there was a point where we had to make the link and say because of the contamination of the blood supply many of the hemophiliacs in Canada became infected. These are the statistics and we are asking the federal government for financial assistance, and you can do your part by signing your name and sending this off. So, by approaching the donor list and asking them to do this, we were not approaching any specific person. It was totally anonymous. Some people signed their full names, others signed just a first name." The idea was to let the government know that there were people out there who were paying attention, and were concerned.

Many hemophiliacs were afraid of making the campaign a public issue. David Page wanted to bring the story out into the open, but not many people were prepared to take the chance. "We needed individuals who were ready to speak out openly and we didn't have any, or very many," he recalls. "I did find a couple of brothers in Quebec who were well-spoken and knowledgeable and who had a story that would get public attention and sympathy. They got quite a bit of play in the media in late 1989 at a critical time. In the English media I don't think we had much coverage at all, and we certainly didn't have anyone who was ready to put their name forward."

Following the 1988 election, Jake Epp was replaced in the health portfolio by Perrin Beatty. Although Epp had turned over the dossier to Greg Smith of his department for further research, the CHS found it was back to square one. Beatty, however, signalled his awareness of the issue in his first speech as health minister, two days after his appointment. But the AIDS-related death on January 9, 1989, of the Catastrophe Relief Committee's honorary chairman, Bob Gibson, was a reminder of the urgency. A meeting was held with Beatty in late winter of 1989.

At the same time as the hemophiliacs' campaign was on, the War Amputees had been clamouring for compensation for the people who had been affected by another health scandal two decades before in the thalidomide affair. The approaches of the two groups were quite different, although there was a recognition that the CHS might have to resort to a public campaign.

"As they were very public and vociferous, we tried to be low-key and work in a very diplomatic way. The other group staged protests and marches and put out documents before the minister could see them, and those kinds of things," says Woloschuk. "We carried on an extensive lobbying of cabinet ministers, including key members of the planning and priorities committee [of cabinet] to get their support. We tried to keep the opposition informed of our status and the kinds of responses we were getting. They kept chomping at the bit waiting to get the okay from us to ask questions in the House. We really didn't want to do that because we kept making progress."

David Page and another member met with Sheila Copps, then Liberal health critic, to get her backing. "When we walked in, she was against the idea of compensation. We sat down with her for an hour and explained what had happened and we walked out with her support. Our approach was to make it an all-party, non-confrontational kind of thing. Nobody had said no to us."

Woloschuk, a member of the Progressive Conservative Party, also attended a convention as a party delegate and met as many politicians as she could. "I said to them: 'Remember that letter you got from the

Hemophilia Society about compensation or catastrophe relief? Well, I'm the person who wrote the letter.'"

Page recalls going with Woloschuk to private Conservative Party cocktail parties and meeting Beatty and other ministers. While Woloschuk used her party connections, Page just crashed the events. He did the same at an international AIDS conference in Montreal in 1989. The message to Beatty was, Remember us? We're going to meet you at every opportunity and we're not going to stop.

There were other, less traditional means of getting through. In 1989, French hemophiliacs blew up the car of Michel Garetta, the government official who was jailed later for his part in that country's blood scandal. A newspaper clipping was sent to Beatty on the bombing along with a letter. "There were appropriate comments that this was not our way but we had to find a solution to this problem because people are really upset," says Page.

A key period was March and April 1989. After the meeting with Beatty, Woloschuk wrote the minister March 23 to warn that many members were becoming frustrated and restless. "I don't know how much longer this explosive issue can be contained," she said. "Our own human and financial resources are becoming seriously strained." There was word that hemophiliacs in Montreal and Calgary were preparing to launch lawsuits. Dr. John Furesz, director of the Bureau of Biologics, begged the CHS in April to reassure its members that the new breed of blood products, in use exclusively for nine months, were safe.

A Decima telephone survey commissioned by the CHS had found two-thirds of Canadians favoured compensation for hemophiliacs who contract AIDS through tainted blood. A majority said the federal government should pay up; smaller groups said insurers, the distributors of blood, the provinces, or all of the above, should bear responsibility. An April 11 meeting with federal officials was positive, although Dr. A. J. Liston, assistant deputy minister, warned the CHS not to focus on government responsibility for blood product safety when making its claim. "The government should then be obliged to refute such allegations," a CHS summary quotes him as saying. Another federal official, policy analyst Greg Smith, suggested the CHS should "avoid statements that could call into question the adequacy of our country's various welfare systems in taking care of the needs of their citizens." The uniqueness of the case and the notion of "compassionate responsibility" should be emphasized, the officials said.

The cause may have been helped along by an article in the *Ottawa Law Review* in 1989 by Sanda Rodgers, then vice-dean of the Common Law Section at the University of Ottawa. Rodgers had written on liability for blood-related injuries and said those harmed by blood products had a good case for compensation other than that which might be awarded through the courts. "In my view, compensation for those injured by blood products is compelled by our moral obligation towards the recipients of Canadian blood products, where regulation and funding for the production of these products is significantly government-controlled," Rodgers wrote.

Beatty may have been getting similar advice from the Justice Department. Whatever the case, he was more personally receptive to the notion of financial assistance than his predecessor. Within two or three months of the meeting, Beatty sent a letter saying he was committed to the principle, but the details had to be worked out. At the end of October, CHS representatives were called to Ottawa and told a financial offer would be made, but drug benefits and spousal benefits would not be paid. The amount was still left open. The Society had proposed a graded system of benefits based on age, marital status, and whether there were children to support, but the federal officials rejected that idea. With the existing concern about the Charter of Rights, the federal government decided it would be discriminatory to offer different packages to different people.

"We had no idea how much money was going to be offered. In fact, we didn't know until the day the announcement was made," recalls Woloschuk. "There was no negotiating with the government; that was their decision. It was up to us to either recommend it to the membership or to tell them to reject it, or let them make their own decision."

The announcement was delayed by two events. Beatty wanted to talk with his provincial counterparts near the end of November to invite them to participate. Woloschuk remembers that she went to a meeting in Prince Edward Island to talk with Wayne Cheverie, then P.E.I.'s health minister and chairman of the provincial ministers' council. The provinces were upset.

"Essentially, the message was: the federal government isn't going to tell us what we should be doing, and we're certainly not going to participate in this project. It was pretty adversarial."

Page says provincial ministers complained the federal government was acting unilaterally. But Beatty had asked them to get involved months before and the provinces had not been interested. "This was really bad news for us," says Page. "We could see we wouldn't get a global settlement, only partial, and then we'd have to deal with ten different provinces. We'd had enough trouble mounting a campaign against one government, with all the resources of the Society."

A second reason for delay was the sudden interest at the Red Cross, after Beatty's announcement, in climbing aboard. To receive the federal offer, recipients would have to sign a waiver that they would not sue the federal government. "At the last minute, the Red Cross wanted to be included on that waiver," says Woloschuk. "They didn't want to have any part in the discussions up until that point, but they wanted to be in on the waiver so nobody could sue the Red Cross. We talked about this and said we're not going to delay this so the Red Cross can get on the bandwagon. If they are on the bandwagon, they'd better ante up. So we just went ahead with the announcement without having the Red Cross on the waiver." Page says a very strong letter was sent to the government that the CHS would not agree to the Red Cross being included.

Woloschuk remembers meeting Roger Perrault of the Red Cross around the summer or early fall of 1989. "I came away from that meeting feeling that he didn't consider the Hemophilia Society a force to be reckoned with. It was a kind of arrogance, like 'Who's this

Mrs. Windsor coming here? Who are you?' It was quite interesting. I don't think I had a lot of credibility in his eyes."

Perrault may have had his eyes opened a little later that fall. The Red Cross was definitely concerned about their liability in the tainted blood affair. Some who had received bad blood had already investigated legal actions. At the November 1989 meeting of the advisory group to the Canadian Blood Committee, Perrault asked if the federal program would halt current litigation. Bill Mindell, the CHS representative, mentioned the waiver that would let the federal government off the hook. The minutes say Mindell "noted that it may be possible to receive extraordinary assistance and yet sue the Canadian Red Cross Society." Later in the meeting, Perrault addressed events that had set a rumour flying that the Red Cross was getting out of the blood business. Because of its "potential liability for blood-related HIV infection," the Red Cross board had considered separating the Blood Transfusion Service from other activities, he said.

That meeting was told that Liston, the assistant deputy minister for Health Protection, had written Woloschuk to say there would be a favourable response to the request for extraordinary assistance. It was also expected that 350 persons infected through blood transfusions would be added to an estimated 950 contaminated hemophiliacs eligible for compensation.

In the fall of 1988, when Epp was still minister, the compensation negotiations had come to the attention of a small group in Calgary who had become HIV-infected after surgery. They wrote Epp to request that they be included if awards were made to recipients of bad blood. When Beatty took over, he assured them that their case would receive serious consideration in any assistance plan that was set up. In the spring of 1989, Greg Smith was dispatched to Calgary to meet with the group.

Spreading word about financial assistance to the post-operative victims of bad blood proved to be a chore, especially since some had no idea they were infected. British Columbia's provincial AIDS committee expressed concern in 1990, for example, that while hemophiliacs attending clinics regularly would know their blood was tainted, blood-transfused people were poorly informed. The government extended its deadline for applications to take notice of those situations.

In one extreme case, a man in his fifties from Simcoe, Ontario, with no support group in his community, didn't know until 1993 that there was a federal assistance plan. He was delivering pizzas for a living.

On December 14, 1989, Beatty made the announcement of the federal extraordinary assistance package in the Commons. It provided for a total of $120,000 for each infected individual in equal instalments spread over four years. The first payment would be made, once waivers were signed, in April 1990.

At the joint news conference following Beatty's statement, Health officials did not know what the CHS would do. "They weren't sure whether we were going to support it, or speak kindly of it, or totally blast it," says Woloschuk. "There was no way I was going to thumb my nose at it. From the calls we had from the membership, they were quite pleased because they had expected nothing."

The amount was a little better than a third of what the CHS had wanted. The federal government proposed that the provinces augment the compensation.

Looking back, Woloschuk says the defining moment was the first meeting with Beatty. "The relationship that was established between himself and the Hemophilia Society at that point was the decisive moment. He listened to the stories that David Page and I told, very cheerfully and compassionately. I think he had had personal experience with a person with HIV and that it was his attitude that carried it forward."

Occasionally Woloschuk is asked about the signposts on the way to a successful resolution. They couldn't be seen at the time, she says. It's only now in looking back that they can be identified. Given the political and economic climate of the day, when government spending was being trimmed in many areas, she feels the assistance was a huge accomplishment. "The door had been opened and the groundwork had been laid."

Page says the talks with the government were not true negotiations in the sense of union-employer bargaining. The Society really had little clout. "All we had was a just cause. We started out with no expectations at all that we'd get a dime."

Around the time the Hemophilia Society was putting its case together in 1987, a task force headed by Robert Prichard, then dean of law at the University of Toronto, had started hearings into the question of liability and compensation for "victims of misadventure within the health care system." The examination of the issue was prompted by a sharp rise in Canadian medical malpractice suits in the previous decade. No one was happy with the situation but the lawyers. Doctors were complaining about liability insurance costs of $200 million, and it was estimated that only 10 per cent of victims legitimately entitled to compensation received anything. The task force was tending towards a no-fault type of compensation for injured parties as an alternative to the costly and time-consuming legal process. A report was expected in a few months. At a meeting of the advisory group to the Canadian Blood Committee in October 1988, it was suggested that hemophiliacs who had seroconverted could be covered under a fund that might be established to cover such situations. When the CHS Catastrophe Relief team met with federal officials, they put the idea on the table.

"It was nothing formal," says David Page today. "We brought it to the talks." The idea was modelled on a Quebec government fund that exists to indemnify parents and provide support in caring for children who have severe reactions to vaccines and become handicapped. "Cases which are no fault of anybody, just an allergic reaction to a vaccine that is unpredictable," says Page.

"When we talked to Greg Smith and the deputy ministers, that was on the table and they seemed to be quite open to having a kind of pharmaceutical misadventure fund." The fund could have applied to cases such as HIV-infected hemophiliacs, thalidomide victims, and the most recent round of infection, hepatitis C. Pharmaceutical companies and governments could make contributions to the fund, says Page. Premiums would rise if something went wrong, providing an incentive for safety. A similar fund was employed in Germany to pay benefits to that country's HIV-positive hemophiliacs.

Page says no action was taken, no promise made, nothing was ever put on paper, and it was not raised at the federal ministerial level. When Quebec hemophiliacs negotiated with their provincial government in the 1990s, however, they raised the subject again.

"When we met with the Quebec government, the ministers there were open to that kind of deal," says Page, who is from Quebec City. "It quickly became evident that was a very big issue. We would have to wait for a long time and we wanted to deal with the hemophilia issue. We wanted to get the thing settled, so it was done independently of any other misadventure scheme."

Bob Pedersen says there had been an "inkling" in the late 1980s the federal government might move in the direction of a fund that could be used where there was no immediately assessable blame and litigation was not a solution. "The simple fact is we live in a world that's motivated by money. If the government and the insurers know they are going to have to spend money, you take care of the system," he says. "You don't want to spend money, so you put in safeguards to ensure that you minimize your costs. But they're medical safeguards. What you have now safeguarding our medical situation is financial safeguards. It's a terrible conflict."

As it turned out, Prichard's report to deputy ministers at the various levels of government was not presented until June 1, 1990. That was after the extraordinary assistance program had begun. Prichard did recommend the compensation fund could be used for future victims of tainted blood, but said he was not making recommendations for those who suffered injury prior to the report. Still, the idea of a medical misadventure fund awaits consideration by future politicians and bureaucrats.

PAT O'CONNOR

Pat O'Connor, a businessman in his early thirties from Cornwall, Ontario, decided to speak out publicly about HIV and AIDS after being appalled at the treatment AIDS victims received in hospitals.

A mild Factor IX hemophiliac, Pat rarely received blood products. But in 1983, when he broke his ankle and had to have pins put in, he needed transfusions. Then, in 1985, his wedding day was rudely interrupted; he had his appendix removed and again needed transfusions. He prefers to think he was infected in 1985 — that would mean the virus has had less time to run its course.

Pat, who once managed truck stops with his wife, Cathy, along Highway 401, is an athletic man who enjoys sports. He admits that he once held homophobic feelings but that having HIV has changed his mind. In fact, it was indignation over how he was treated in a Kingston hospital that led him to go public and challenge the attitudes that people, even in the medical profession, hold towards those with HIV and AIDS.

Six months after his appendix operation, there was a lot of talk in the hemophilia community about the numbers of people who had been infected with HIV. Pat and Cathy were living in Bowmanville, just east of Toronto, and he decided to have his blood checked. His doctor had never dealt with HIV or AIDS before. When preliminary results came back, the doctor told him he had been negative. The happy couple went out to dinner to celebrate.

A backup test, however, reversed the happy news. Pat went to see the doctor alone and didn't tell Cathy about his appointment. The doctor told him he had AIDS.

"I pretty well left that office thinking I was going to die in a year or so," says Pat. "I remember having to go and pick up some Cheez Whiz. The store was only two minutes away. By the time I got there I was terrified, walking around the grocery store thinking about what all these people would do if they knew I had AIDS. Cathy came home from work that night and found me quite drunk."

The O'Connors moved to Cornwall soon after to manage the Fifth Wheel truck stop there. They also bought a couple of submarine sandwich stands in the town along the St. Lawrence, southeast of Ottawa. For his HIV clinic appointments, however, Pat preferred the anonymity of Kingston, a two-hour drive west. In 1990, suffering from headaches and with his T-cell count dropping, Pat was hospitalized overnight in Kingston.

"I was treated very badly at the hospital," Pat recalls. "They had a big Biohazard sign on the outside of my door, and the first night nobody came in to see me. I got into my room at 5 p.m. and went to sleep and somebody brought in my meal and left it on the table, didn't wake me up. For the whole night, nobody came in to check, say 'Hi, here's your water jug.' Anything.

"I was treated like a leper — that's the only way I could explain it. It was degrading and intimidating. The doctor said, 'Oh, you're treated well — because you're a hemophiliac, you're an innocent victim. You're treated better than anyone else in here.'

"And that's when I wondered, if I'm treated 'well' and I feel like this, what about all these other people down the hall — how are they being treated and how do they feel? That's when I decided I'd better go out and start talking about it."

O'Connor was surprised at the ignorance even doctors and nurses in a teaching hospital had about HIV. Fears abounded, but sometimes it wasn't fear that kept them away.

"The nurses on the floor weren't afraid to come into the room because they might catch something. The big thing was they didn't know what to say to me, so they avoided my room. But at the same time they never thought about what that was doing to me up here." He taps his head.

"I just remember that when a nurse came in and held my hand or touched my arm, it made me feel a lot better. It still does when anybody touches me, because you know they're not afraid of you."

* * *

Pat's first talks were made at that hospital. He spoke to the housekeeping staff and to nurses. Then he began speaking at other hospitals and at nurses' colleges. At first, he stayed well away from Cornwall, but then he started giving talks in Brockville, about halfway between Kingston and his home town.

"For a long time I was terrified I was going to run into somebody from Cornwall. But then I started looking at our own community, and AIDS wasn't talked about there. It was like it never existed."

There were rumours to deal with. Because of his headaches, a side-effect of the drug AZT and the constant stress, Pat was having increasing difficulty doing his job. He had always been energetic, but now he had to lie down for a rest every day at noon.

"I was pretty screwed up in my head, because you take two AZT pills in the morning and you are already starting to have a headache by noon, and then you have to take two more. Sometimes I'd look out my office window and say, What the hell am I doing here? I'm going home to sleep.

Pat believed he would be fired if this continued, so he explained to the company president what was happening. "He eased me out of the company really slowly and quietly. He sort of let on I was going to run my own businesses, paid me a year's salary, and carried my benefits. I was quite lucky."

Meanwhile, Cathy was working crazy hours trying to keep the submarine stands going. Finally, the O'Connors put the businesses up for sale.

"My dad wondered what the hell was going on. My parents lived out in Penticton, in the Okanagan — they had retired there. That was one reason I'd never told them. I knew if I told them they'd end up back here. He called and was upset with me, so the next day I jumped on a plane to go out to tell them. I never realized until after I told them that any parent's biggest fear is losing one of their kids."

Pat and Cathy, who tests HIV-negative, had already told a few select friends. Four of them learned about Pat's HIV status at a fondue party shortly after the O'Connors had returned to Cornwall. After three or four bottles of wine, the bad news was broached. The news was devastating, but the two couples remain friends with the O'Connors. Pat says his friends have been great: "I just can't explain how much they've been behind me, and helped me when I needed to talk."

Once Pat was giving his talks, the pressure to go public mounted. There was a need for public education about HIV and AIDS, but the biggest need was for Cathy and Pat to lift the burden of secrecy.

"We had to stop telling lies. Life was just too stressful, and it wasn't helping my health any. When I finally did go public, it was the most weight ever lifted off me after five years living in fear, hiding it."

Pat contacted the Cornwall daily newspaper — the *Standard-Freeholder* — in September 1991, and they did a front-page story and a full page inside on the O'Connors, HIV, and AIDS. The Saturday that the stories were published, Pat and Cathy were out of town.

"When we got home on Sunday, the answering machine was jammed with people calling, most of them saying, 'God bless,' 'Good luck,' or 'Glad you did it.' It was all positive stuff."

Going public in his home town of about 46,000 allowed Pat to speak out there now. He began writing a column on living with HIV and AIDS in the newspaper. He found there were quite a few infected people in the community who had never had a focal point before. He believes that because he is a hemophiliac, it is easier for him to speak out.

"The message to get across is that this is not a gay thing. Sure, I'm Pat the Hemophiliac. But would people treat me the same if I was Pat the Gay, or Pat the Drug User? I still tend to think not, and I realized that when I started public speaking. Unfortunately, a hemophiliac is a good person to get the message across about AIDS. You can get up in front of a hundred people and say: 'I'm Pat, I'm a hemophiliac, I'm married, and I got HIV from blood,' and you've got everybody's attention."

Pat has worked with a support group for AIDS in Cornwall since revealing his status. "A lot of them are dead now. A lot of them can't eat properly. They might need drugs, and they can't afford them." On several occasions, he spoke on panels in Kingston with two gay men. One was a young man who was thrown out of his home as a teenager when he revealed his infection to his parents. The other was a man in his fifties who was on his deathbed four times, with funeral arrangements made but kept coming back for more panel discussions. Both died within a week of each other in the fall of 1993. Their deaths shook Pat.

Pat tries not to be angry over what has happened to himself and others. After an initial burst of rage when he found out he was infected, he saw that anger as a waste of energy. But he admits he has been angry again recently as more facts about what happened to the blood supply became public knowledge. He was also upset when he attended a youth retreat in Vancouver sponsored by the Canadian Hemophilia Society.

"I was one of the oldest guys there. I got angry when I saw teenagers twelve and thirteen, sixteen, eighteen years old. When I was there listening to those kids — about what they were afraid of, the relationship problem, marriage, all the things I had already done and I already had — I felt lucky. So my anger was more about how they got it."

He's also concerned about what he sees as the attention given the sick person in a partnership, while the other partner is ignored. "For a long time, all the attention went to me. It happens to gay couples, too. And then one day a few years ago we were at the clinic in Kingston, and Cathy was in talking to the social worker. She said, 'How are you?' and Cathy started shaking; she was ready to have a nervous breakdown. She was a mess because nobody paid attention to her health and she's the one living with me. That isn't easy because of mood swings through the years and depression, and worrying about losing her husband. And that's when we started looking after Cathy."

Pat says a lot of people ask why Cathy would stay with him. "You have to wonder what kinds of relationships these people have. Would you leave your wife if she came home and said 'I have cancer'?"

Chapter 13

TEST OF COURAGE

*"They say Christ was killed for thirty pieces of silver, so
taking inflation into account, $30,000 isn't so bad."*
JOHN WILSON, A HEMOPHILIAC, JANUARY 1994

The federal government had told the Hemophilia Society negotiators
that Ottawa had done its part. For more help, Health and Welfare
officials said, go to the provinces.

Perrin Beatty, the federal health minister in 1989, gave his blessing. "I have invited the provinces to do their part in view of their role
in the national blood system," Beatty said. "And I support the Society's
efforts to obtain additional assistance from the provinces."

This was all very well, but the provinces were not in any mood
to bite. Goliath Ottawa may have fallen, but the armies of the
Philistines were now arrayed in the provincial capitals.

"They very steadfastly dug in their heels and one after another
decided they were not going to participate in this," Elaine Woloschuk
recalls. The provinces did agree they would not tax the federal benefits, nor would they use it as part of the means test when infected-blood
victims applied for disability and social security. But that was it.

A strategy meeting attended by national and provincial representatives of the CHS was held during January 1990 in Montreal. At
that point it was believed Ontario would be the key to a settlement,
but that Quebec, with its traditional focus on social measures, might
be expected to show the most sympathy. The theory was that they

would likely have a tougher time with the smaller provinces, but there was hope that a large province would concede that compensation was just and that the provinces had to answer for a role in the disaster, thereby setting a precedent.

The national executives of the CHS wanted out. Despite their recognition that the take-it-or-leave-it federal offer was not all the country's hemophiliacs had hoped for, they felt it was important that the provincial chapters tackle their respective governments.

"This is as far as we can take you," said Woloschuk. "You have to work on this on your own, carrying on lobbying campaigns and things like that. Provincial governments would want to talk to provincial members, and provincial members are better poised to influence their governments than the national ones are."

The gruelling talks with Ottawa had taken a toll. Woloschuk was relieved it was over after spending countless hours and one weekend after another on the project. "I don't think anybody had any inkling of the amount of time used in volunteer and staff hours." Vice-president David Page, the head of the Society's compensation committee, was exhausted. Some of the HIV-positive members who had worked on the committee were dying. The provincial chapters were pretty much on their own.

Page made that clear. "While the national CHS will commit some volunteer and staff time to helping, your chapter resources will have to bear the lion's share of the effort," he wrote. "Be aware that a provincial catastrophe relief campaign will almost certainly require more time and energy on your parts than any project your chapter has ever undertaken."

At that point, the need didn't seem that urgent. Most infected hemophiliacs were excited that compensation, although generally perceived as inadequate, had been wrung from an initially reluctant federal government. The money would give them something for a while at least. Who knew if any of them would be alive by the time the provinces would ante up?

Then fresh troops entered the scene. Among them was John

Plater, a tall red-haired man from Collingwood, Ontario, then barely out of his teens and a university student. Plater is articulate, enthusiastic, and polite. He believed the cause was not only just but winnable. It he had a fault, it may have been that he was too trusting that the other side would see the justice of compensation. Himself HIV-positive, Plater had the makings of a modern-day hero for those who suffered from tainted blood.

He jumped into the fray quickly. Plater met in the spring of 1990 with Elinor Caplan, then health minister in Ontario's Liberal government.

"It was something," Plater recalls. "I remember saying to her: 'This is an honour for a first-year political science student from the University of Toronto to be sitting here with one of the most powerful members of the government discussing issues.'"

Plater's youthful exuberance didn't have an immediate pay-off. Caplan said the subject was being discussed inter-provincially. A meeting would come in the fall.

By September, everything had changed. Bob Rae's New Democrats had won a stunning and unexpected election victory that month, and the game had to begin again.

Caplan's successor was Evelyn Gigantes, a political veteran from Ottawa. Gigantes had missed the inter-provincial conference where compensation had been discussed but met with hemophilia representatives in November.

"We walked in and you immediately realized this was a new government, they were full of this 'How do we govern?' sort of thing. The minister came out and met us in the hallway. It was nice. Elinor Caplan had three or four young men dressed in suits with her, carrying everything and holding everything. Almost like maids.

"It was like going to granny's house. I honestly waited for Evelyn Gigantes to say, 'Do you want cookies?' She ushered us into her office. She took her own notes. And she turned to us and said: 'Well, I guess that's about $250,000 apiece, and you have so many people, so it's going to cost us this much.' We were a little taken aback. It seemed a bit naive on her part. You know, I'm the minister and I can do anything. But we felt great. We didn't sense there was something binding her."

What Plater didn't know, and possibly what Gigantes was not aware of given her newness to the portfolio, was that officials of all the provincial governments had met in September 1990 and settled on a common front — no provincial compensation for blood-transfused victims.

Meanwhile, Plater and his colleagues kept up the lobbying, meeting each member of the cabinet social policy committee. The visit by lawyer James Kreppner, a hemophiliac, to Social Services Minister Zanana Akande led to one of the few lighter moments in what was a grim exercise. After delegates had outlined the whole story of how the blood supply came to be tainted by HIV and what the Society wanted, Akande looked up. "Why didn't they use condoms?" she asked.

"James was ready to jump on the table at her," laughs Plater. "It was like, Is this what we're dealing with?"

Gigantes was replaced in the spring of 1991 by Frances Lankin, and Plater says that was when his optimism disappeared. When the New Democrats won their shocking electoral victory on September 6, 1990, some hemophiliacs had a sense of elation. This was a government that would listen to the aggrieved, they felt. The New Democrats had a reputation for compassion and would recognize the justice in special assistance for tainted blood victims. Their hope was overblown.

Many New Democrats, whose supporters included a large share of the gay population, did not make any distinction between the tragedy that had befallen the homosexual community and that which struck at those who had acquired HIV as a result of bad choices made by publicly accountable officials in charge of the national blood system.

Lankin was one. She noted tersely that government assistance was available to all who suffered from AIDS. Specific groups would not be treated differently. She pointed out the Ontario government had made contributions to the Hemophilia Society. Akande did send a letter confirming that Ontario would exempt the federal compensation paid to tainted blood victims, and their survivors, when social assistance applications were made. This was not enough for those whose blood had been contaminated by transfusions.

Kreppner, one of Hemophilia Ontario's negotiators in the talks with the province, felt Lankin feigned sympathy. "Frances Lankin demonstrated a complete lack of empathy and understanding. She was doing her best to avoid responsibility," Kreppner said in September 1993. "They were never hostile. They would say they could understand and would study the concerns."

Kreppner says the secret of the provincial agreement was never revealed, though some negotiators suspected something was going on. "They led us on. That there was an agreement among the provinces was never relayed to us. They talked to us, but not in good faith."

Lankin continued to hold firm. "I'm not sure we're going to do anything about this," Plater reports her saying. She was more explicit in replies to Saskatchewan New Democrats who had written her, probing Ontario's stance on the issue. "Our government has decided it will not provide additional funding to the specific people who have contracted HIV through the blood supply," she told Chris Axworthy, the NDP representative on the House of Commons sub-committee on health issues, in October 1992.

The closest Lankin came to having second thoughts may have been during a meeting in July 1991 when she was flipping through a package of material the Society had prepared. "Her eyes stuck on something," says Plater. "We think it was the Australian situation — the kid with the lawsuit who won. And the big thing is that it cost $15 million to fight that. We're positive her eyes caught that, and she just said: 'I'm going to review this and meet with you again in a week.'"

The hemophiliacs had agreed to steer away from legal arguments, despite Kreppner's legal training, but they did point out that the mounting number of lawsuits would cost the system dearly, should victims feel compelled to test the courts. "It was good to have someone on the team who knew the law so we couldn't be bluffed," says Kreppner. "I didn't play it up. I was there as an officer of Hemophilia Ontario and the chair of the Society's AIDS advisory committee."

But any hope of a breakthrough was short-lived. Lankin decided in August 1991 not to place the compensation issue before the cabinet. The talks had proven fruitless.

Some victims of the tainted blood were growing desperate. Their T-cell counts, measuring the immune system's ability to fight off attacks, continued to drop while opportunistic infections mounted. Anxiety increased, which didn't do anything to improve their health. Court cases piled up as dozens of the victims, although reluctant to sue, felt there was little choice but to confront governments and the Red Cross in legal battles that might be a pyrrhic victory. There was certainly no shortage of legal advice. Some lawyers suggested class action might be a possibility under Ontario's changing law, to be proclaimed in 1993, others said no chance. Some lawyers advised their clients there was little possibility of winning a suit unless they had a previous negative test. This was an appalling Catch-22. Many — perhaps most — hemophiliacs had been infected by tainted blood before they were first tested for the virus. This was especially true of the severest hemophiliacs, who also had the highest rate of infection. The transfused-blood victims may have had a better case. Often, their contamination could be linked to a few transfusions in a limited time period.

Meanwhile, lawyers were sprouting up like spring flowers. The Ottawa branch of Hemophilia Ontario, which also included many Quebec hemophiliacs who crossed the river for treatment at the city's large hospitals, welcomed two young lawyers from the renowned Toronto firm of Goodman & Goodman.

They had a persuasive pitch and several families signed on, only to find themselves dropped by the firm after thousands of dollars had been spent, in some cases by families that could ill afford the losses. Most hemophiliacs were stung by Goodman & Goodman's decision to drop their case. Whatever the reason, Goodman & Goodman had left a bad taste with many hemophiliacs.

Still, in the light of the immovable provinces, the legal route seemed the only sure way to go. Some plaintiffs intended to carry through their suits to the end; others saw it as a pressure tactic to get the provinces to the negotiating table. It would be expensive and time-consuming for both sides. The worst cases, those of people with families and unable to work, would find the legal route expensive. They needed money *now*, not three or four years down the road after all lawyers had taken their cut and court costs were subtracted. A court victory would cost the tax-paying public, the governments, the Red Cross, the hospitals, and doctors, and perhaps the fractionators. But the plaintiffs themselves might have been hardest hit, even in victory.

Meanwhile, CHS members kept up the pressure. In the fall of 1992, about thirty Ontario victims gathered in a Burlington, Ontario, hotel for a strategy session. The government had closed the doors, and the status quo was not acceptable, said Mark Bulbrook, one of the activists. There was need for lobbying, a media campaign, and other kinds of activist action. When John Plater told a news conference early in 1993 that members had talked of blocking Toronto's Gardiner Expressway during rush hour, or chaining themselves to Premier Bob Rae's front door, or throwing fake (or even real) blood on Health Minister Lankin, he wasn't exaggerating. Though Plater urged the angriest to cool it, all of those possibilities were raised at the Burlington meeting as ways of raising the public profile of compensation.

This angry radicalism was new to Canadian hemophiliacs. For years, hemophiliacs had been passive and almost obsequious in their dealings with politicians, the medical profession, and the blood authorities. There had been widespread respect for doctors, even those with dubious knowledge of hemophilia. Instead of anger for the way many hemophiliacs had been shabbily treated, there was perverse gratitude. That reaction was changing as the horror of the tragedy unfolded. But some CHS members were still fearful that if they stepped too far out of line, doctors and hospitals would refuse to treat them, and agencies like the Red Cross would somehow punish offenders.

Some members of the Burlington group expressed fears that volunteer donors might not give blood to the Red Cross if hemophiliacs kicked up too much of a stink. The publicity might scare the public off.

In late February 1993, Plater was discouraged with the lack of progress. His term as president of Hemophilia Ontario was coming to an end. He felt that he and the Society had failed and wondered aloud at meetings whether it was worth continuing the effort. But somehow he stayed on to lead the provincial compensation team after he turned over the president's chair.

Just when the compensation effort seemed to be stalled, a break-through came in a most unexpected part of Canada. Over time, the perception of where a break in the provincial ranks would occur had changed. Ontario had proven a tough nut to crack. Plater credits James Kreppner with recognizing that a small province might be the first to move. "It's got to be a small place," Plater recalls Kreppner saying.

"Our plan had been to identify the small province that would go easy and then parachute in people to make it happen. We talked about one of the Maritime provinces being the obvious choice. Some-place with next to no one there. Prince Edward Island, for example."

Plater and Kreppner didn't need to develop their idea much further. A couple from Nova Scotia, Janet and Randy Conners, were already making things happen on their own.

George Moody is an affable former school principal, a bespectacled grey-haired man with a sympathetic face who could easily be lost in a crowd. But to the victims of the tainted blood scandal, he comes close to being elevated to sainthood.

Skeptics may say Moody, Nova Scotia's Progressive Conserva-tive health minister until the summer of 1993, was acting out of political desperation. A provincial election was coming up, and the Tory government was on the ropes. Besides all the other problems — scandals, high unemployment — the government was confronted with, there was one issue that was particularly embarrassing and had received national publicity.

This was the case of the Conners family, a husband and wife who were both infected with HIV. Randy was a hemophiliac and Janet had become infected through her husband. The couple also had a son, Gus, entering his teens. Their poignant plight received wide publicity, focusing especially on what was to become of their child when they were no longer around to look after him. Randy had already showed signs of advanced illness.

Moody had been appointed to office in October 1990, a month after provincial health ministers had secretly agreed not to compensate tainted blood victims. He maintained the united front until he met with Randy and Janet.

"I don't think until I had an opportunity to meet Randy and Janet that I really appreciated the need for compensation," Moody said in September 1993. "When I had the meeting and learned about the difficulties, I got to understand what they had to deal with on a day-to-day basis. I didn't feel we had to put them through the welfare system. Compensation wouldn't have been any greater cost to the government. It was unfair that they would have to struggle."

Janet Conners, for her part, knew the family's problems had registered with Moody. She told reporters later she caught a look in Moody's eye and knew then that he would do something.

Moody raised the issue of compensation at a health ministers meeting in British Columbia in January 1993. "Nobody was too interested." But the ministers also knew if one province caved in, it would break the resistance. Moody was already taking heat from his colleagues. He backed off, thinking perhaps the compensation issue could be revisited at the next scheduled health ministers conference in September 1993.

"I knew these were special people," says Moody. "Then I felt if we didn't do something, it wouldn't be achieved in September. On that basis, I took it to the cabinet. It was an easy sell for some, including the premier [Donald Cameron]. Others were a little reluctant."

Moody announced on April 14 that the province would enter into negotiations and it got immediate attention across the country.

Hemophiliacs were suddenly big news, on national television and in the newspapers.

Nova Scotia came up with a proposal. It would provide $30,000 to each victim directly or indirectly infected by the blood supply for life, provide AIDS drugs free, include $50,000 in life insurance, $5,000 for funeral expenses, and four years of post-secondary education for children and care-giving spouses.

Moody's decision was like the breakup of a log jam, encouraging blood-transfusion victims in the other provinces to try harder. Ontario's new health minister, Ruth Grier, said she would review her policy and talk things over with the other provinces. Grier pronounced herself in sympathy with the victims and agreed to make a recommendation to her cabinet colleagues.

"Governments in the past did not adopt policies that protected people who received blood," Grier told the *Globe and Mail.*

Plater and others who had dealt with the Ontario ministry were pleasantly surprised that Grier seemed more open. Grier, for good reason, seemed to have a more personal stake in the issue of blood safety and compensation. At one meeting, she talked about her late husband's surgery and how she took him to be tested afterwards.

And personality mattered, one member of the compensation committee said later, contrasting Grier with Frances Lankin. The new minister seemed genuinely sympathetic. It appeared something significant would happen in Ontario.

British Columbia minister Elizabeth Cull, also a New Democrat, said a thoughtful response was required.

Quebec was the next province to come up with an offer, but the 260 victims in that province were furious at its limited scope. Health Minister Marc-Yvan Côté said the compensation fund would be $10 million and the money distributed following a means test. The proposal reinforced the anger of the victims.

Bad blood recipients, encouraged by the spreading response but still fearful that the Nova Scotia offer would be isolated, stepped up their lobbying. Legislatures and a meeting of deputy ministers in Ottawa were picketed.

Saskatchewan was one of the holdouts. Early in June 1993, Lorne Calvert, associate minister of health, wrote a letter to Craig Wright, the provincial CHS president, that is a classic in terms of abdication of responsibility. In a four-paragraph letter, Calvert managed to say twice that the federal government was legally on the hook and the province was not.

He also noted the Commons sub-committee on health issues had called on Ottawa to reassess the adequacy of the four-year compensation package it had started in 1993. "This is indeed encouraging," Calvert said, adding that he agreed with the recommendation because of the federal regulatory responsibility. He conveniently ignored the recommendation by the same committee that Ottawa "urge and assist" the provinces and territories to put together their own package to complement the federal payout. "The provincial government does not have the resources required to compensate all persons in tragic circumstances," Calvert wrote.

George Moody's unrepentant gesture, while publicly applauded, did not save the doomed Cameron government from electoral disaster. It went down in a May election, like a vessel hitting bottom on the jagged rocks of Nova Scotia. But Moody won his riding. And the succeeding Liberal government was not about to reverse the settlement.

John Plater says Moody should be given credit. "George took it to heart. It became his issue. He made it happen."

Does Moody have any regrets in retrospect?

"I regret maybe that we didn't do it a bit sooner," he said reflectively, after the other nine provinces had come up with their own offers.

Usually, he said, when you make a move like that someone will complain. "But I haven't had anyone come to me and say that was a bad decision."

Although the Nova Scotia offer set the stage for a settlement in the rest of Canada, the struggle in the other nine provinces and two territories was not finished. Meetings took place throughout the spring and summer of 1993 and in August a preliminary offer was made by provincial deputy ministers, which included $30,000 a year for four years for those directly infected, survivors benefits for spouses and children, and the signing of a comprehensive waiver.

Ontario CHS president Tom Alloway said in a letter to Grier that the annual payments should be for life. "We could never recommend to our members any package that did not contain a lifetime commitment to the affected individuals. The problem with time-limited payments is that some people would inevitably face severe financial hardship at the very end of their lives when they are least able to look after themselves."

Alloway also warned that anger against the Red Cross ran high in the hemophilia and blood-transfused groups. Unless the Red Cross contributed "very substantially," governments should avoid including the agency in the waiver, Alloway added. "Emotional feeling against the Red Cross is very strong, and the government should not underestimate the role which emotion may play in determining whether people who are suing will accept any package."

With the renewed input from the victims, the deputy ministers came up with an assistance package on September 15, 1993, worth "well over" $130 million. The plan, entitled the Multi-Provincial Territorial Assistance Program, offered $30,000 annually for life for those directly infected through blood. It included a payment upon enrolment in the program and four years of benefits for surviving spouses and children. At the same time, an inquiry into the blood system was announced. Ontario Judge Horace Krever was later named to conduct the inquiry.

There were significant shortcomings to the program. Spouses or children infected indirectly by the recipient of bad blood would not get the $30,000 annual payment. Parents or other care-givers who may have given up jobs to look after their dying relatives got nothing. The assistance was not indexed to inflation, meaning that those who were not yet AIDS-symptomatic would in reality have less money to deal with their needs down the road. There was nothing to cover the heavy costs of drugs and medical equipment needed by those fighting off the ravages of HIV-AIDS infection. This was a major disappointment. Hemophilia Ontario negotiators, at least, say they were told during talks that costs of drugs needed to fight off AIDS-related infection would be covered by a drug plan for all sufferers from the syndrome. This promise appeared to fade as the March 15, 1994, deadline for the package neared, but by December, Premier Bob Rae had resurrected it. Though the future of his government was uncertain, he pledged that a comprehensive drug plan would be put into effect in 1995.

There are instances, possibly widespread, in which the failure to provide a comprehensive drug plan could cost governments more than they'd save. Kreppner told the Krever inquiry that one time when he was hospitalized with pneumonia he wanted to get a drug called Mepron, which is not on the officially approved list. Mepron costs $800 for a month's supply, but with this drug he could have gone home instead of occupying an expensive hospital bed and having to take another drug intravenously. Kreppner got approval for Mepron through an emergency release, but in the meantime filled a hospital bed for two weeks, costing far more than the desired drug.

The assistance plan also provided that if a cure came, the payments stopped, with no provision for training so people could re-enter — or enter for the first time, in many cases — the labour market. And those who qualified but had been late receiving the federal assistance package would have to exhaust their claim on Ottawa before they could get compensation from the provincial one.

Few of the 1,000 victims of tainted blood were pleased by the plan. When Ontario's assistant deputy health minister, Michael Ennis, and Phil Dresch of the Canadian Blood Agency appeared at a meeting in Toronto in late October to clarify the package, they must have thought they'd stepped into a lion's den. They faced three hours of one enraged question and denunciation after another. When Ennis looked away to reply to one poignant question, a woman who had lost her sister demanded he look at her when he responded. The mood was angry and defiant.

Evidently, the Red Cross and the four manufacturers of blood products used in Canada in the mid-1980s — and their insurers — thought they'd seen a deal emerging that would get them off the hook. They leapt on the assistance bandwagon, too. Unlike the rebuff it had received at the time of the federal assistance program, this time the Red Cross was successful in clambering aboard. When the package emerged in final form in early December 1993, it raised the initial enrolment payment to $22,000 from $20,000, a modest increase hardly enough to cover a few months' supply of drugs. Surviving spouses fared better — they would now get five years of payments of $20,000 annually and children would receive $4,000 each for five years.

The new proposal was certainly a better deal for the provinces, whose Canadian Blood Agency was to administer the program. While the total cost was to rise to $151 million, the provincial share now dropped to $109 million, while the blood-fractionating companies kicked in $42 million.

There was widespread dissatisfaction with the package among those who had suffered from tainted blood. What really angered them was that in order to receive the package, they were compelled to sign, by March 15, 1994, a complex twenty-four-page waiver agreeing to drop all legal action that might have been started. As predicted by Alloway, many recipients wanted the Red Cross and other parties left out of the waiver. There was widespread feeling that the Red Cross and pharmaceutical manufacturers had come aboard late, tossed in what for most victims would be a pittance more, and expected to be released. Worse, for many people, was that they were being compelled to lie to get the assistance. They were forced to agree that they were not under duress and their legal advisors had to shut their mouths and play along with the falsehood. There was an inherent contradiction in the so-called assistance — sign or get nothing, or undertake costly and lengthy court action. And, by the way, agree that there was no compulsion.

Particularly galling was the fact that they would be forced to decide before the Krever inquiry made any report on the events of the 1980s, that is, before any determination was made of how the system had failed to protect the victims. There were also court cases that might have shed some light on the options, and it was believed these would not be settled before March 15. But most people felt they did not have the financial ability or the health to pursue recourse in the courts. They needed the money now, so they signed up by the hundreds.

Ed Kubin of Lorette, Manitoba, was one of those who was angry. "It's going to place a tremendous amount of stress on hemophiliacs down the line," Kubin said in early March 1994, about a week before the deadline. "We're having a shotgun put to our heads. We're in no position to fight back. To fight would take five to seven years of litigation and we have no way of earning money. That contract is nothing more than a bunch of bullies ganging up on us."

Many people held back, however, waiting for the result of court cases before deciding whether to accept the package or to proceed with their own court action.

The class action option, only made legal in Ontario on January 1, 1993, was an attractive possibility to some. A statement of claim was served on the Red Cross by the London, Ontario, firm of Siskind, Cromarty, Ivey and Dowler on November 15 but could not be issued against the Ontario government because of a requirement for sixty days' notice before suing the province. The March 15 deadline would be close at hand before any decision was made by the judge on whether the action could go ahead.

The class-action decision came sooner than most expected and it was not good for the victims of tainted blood. Judge Robert Montgomery said the claims were of an individual nature and could not be considered as a class. Furthermore, he said, transmission through blood is the "least common means by which HIV is transmitted." Montgomery's statement is extremely misleading. While blood transfusions may account for fewer HIV-AIDS cases than homosexual sex, intravenous drug use, or even heterosexual relations, the likelihood of infection through contaminated blood is extremely high per exposure. For hemophiliacs, at least, infection through blood products was the most common means of transmission — surely a fact that sets them apart as a class. Physicians point out that infection through tainted blood products is the most efficient way to transmit the virus, with an infection rate of greater than 90 per cent from a single exposure to bad blood.

One has to speculate that the suit failed in part because of the choice of the representative plaintiff. She was a Texas resident who came to Ontario for surgery in 1983 and was infected through transfusion, hardly a typical case. However, it was too late at that point to mount a new case or to appeal. The notion of class action died, and those who had counted on it leaned more heavily towards signing the waiver.

Many people were waiting for the case of Rochelle Pittman to be settled, too. That judgment was made on March 14, a day before the infamous deadline.

But the Pittman case did not provide any comfort to those still considering at the last minute whether to pursue lawsuits. Judge Susan Lang said the Red Cross was not negligent in 1984 in its efforts to protect the blood. Worse for the hopeful victims of contaminated blood, Lang stated the Pittman case could not be applied generally to other cases of transfusion-related AIDS.

"It is crucial that the defendants' actions in the 1980s not be judged with the benefit of 1993 information, knowledge, and by hindsight," Lang wrote. "To do so might comfort some by providing scapegoats to blame for the appalling suffering caused by this disease. But this would not be just."

Douglas Lindores, the Red Cross secretary-general, seized on that comment. It gave him "pleasure," a Red Cross news release said, "that the judge's decision confirmed that the Red Cross had acted responsibly to safeguard the Canadian blood supply from the threat of HIV during the scientifically turbulent 1980s."

Most of those still waiting gave up and signed the waiver.

* * *

The process of seeking the meagre compensation took a heavy emotional toll on all those involved, and on those who watched from the sidelines. A debt is owed by all Canadians to those dedicated people. Without them, there would likely not have been any further assistance, and no national inquiry into what went wrong in the blood system. Canada's courts might have been tied up with lawsuits for years, and governments and the Red Cross might have avoided having their activities scrutinized.

The hemophilia and blood-infected communities grieved on September 13, 1994, when Randy Conners passed away. Who can forget the haunting image of a wheelchair-bound Conners, his ravaged face covered by a full beard, waving his finger and hoarsely whispering the question we all want the answer to: "Who done it?"

After his long and valiant fight on the compensation committee, John Plater struggled to control his emotions when he appeared before Judge Krever's inquiry into the blood system in March 1994.

Plater explained he was not angry at the beginning of the process, but he was frustrated at how long it took to get anything accomplished. So many of those infected were gone now and would not benefit from the assistance.

"It will never go away for us," he said, choked up. "But for goodness' sake, it's never to happen again!"

EVA BLAIKIE

When she was seventy-eight years old, Eva Blaikie had to fight to be admitted into a seniors' nursing home.

Although Eva and her daughter Karla remained anonymous throughout the fight, that battle had to be acted out in the public media before authorities were forced to find a suitable place for the ailing, aging woman.

The black mark against Eva Blaikie was that she had AIDS, acquired through a blood transfusion given during an operation in Truro, Nova

Scotia, in February 1985. Like many others infected by contaminated blood, she did not learn from her own family doctor what had happened. Six people may have received the same bad blood at that Truro hospital; only three have been traced by the Red Cross.

Eva was badly arthritic. After her first operation, she went to live with Karla and her family in Dartmouth. Doctors at Camp Hill Hospital in Halifax, where she was in a day program, decided then she needed a total knee replacement.

About ten days after the knee surgery, Karla remembers, one of the doctors called her. "He was very angry. He said I should have told him about my mother's blood problem. I didn't know what he was talking about."

The family doctor admitted later to Karla that he knew Eva was HIV-positive but did not want to tell her. He didn't think it would be a problem. Eva was a widow of advancing age, and nobody would ever have to know what was wrong, he assumed. She told Karla later that it had been rumoured something had gone terribly wrong with the blood at the Colchester Regional Hospital in Truro, but she never thought it involved her.

Eva avoided the issue in the first year she was infected. But Karla, after confirming the test results, started preparing the family for the inevitable.

Some friends and business acquaintances were less than supportive. One friend called up the morning after she was told. "I hate to tell you this, but we can't see you any more," Karla recalls. Another threatened to have her child moved from the class if Karla's son, Eva's grandchild, was in the same room. "To know your kids are going to be hurt, that's the hardest part," Karla says today. Her husband, Bryan, had just launched his dream, a small food business. When Eva got AIDS, he just closed it down.

Life became extremely difficult for Karla, who was a registered nurse working part-time in the Northwood Centre, a seniors' home. Eva would have bouts of illness, sometimes diarrhea that would go on for weeks. Coping with the illness became a strain on the whole family. Karla couldn't get help, either. Homemakers would refuse to come when they heard Eva had AIDS. When her mother was severely ill, Karla would have her taken to Halifax's Victoria General Hospital, where she was given minimal care. Once, when she called an ambulance, the attendants almost dropped her mother when she told them Eva had AIDS. They apologized, Karla says. "They had made a bet between them that no one would ever be honest about AIDS. They said they would never have picked out my mother as an AIDS victim."

In the AIDS wing of the Victoria General, Eva received good care but was something of a curiosity. "There was nobody else her age that she knew had this," says her son David, who lives in Manotick, Ontario.

"She was surrounded by young men who were dying of AIDS. They weren't old women like her. You would see them go up and down the corridor, and they would meet their parents and their sisters and brothers. It was really a poignant thing to see. And yet it wasn't all sad there. People were able to laugh and make jokes and go on in their own way with their lives, and she was part of it that way."

"She was totally shameless," says Karla. " 'I didn't get it how you think I did,' she'd say to them."

When she returned home, the need for constant attention became overwhelming. Karla tried to get her mother admitted to several nursing homes. As soon as she mentioned Eva was an HIV carrier, she was rejected.

Finally, a sympathetic doctor suggested she go to the media. That was a critical decision. At first opposed to playing out the case in the media, Bryan agreed that Karla could take that course but he would never live in the province of Nova Scotia again.

"He was sick and tired of telling anyone," Karla says. "Every time he did, another door would close in his face. He wanted a new start." Bryan moved to New Brunswick and for about nine months they were apart, although they visited back and forth. Meanwhile, Karla put the Dartmouth house up for sale.

David Blaikie was among those caught off-guard by the media publicity. "I was at home one night," he recalled recently. "I was watching the news, and this story came on about an elderly Nova Scotia woman with AIDS. I could see it showing her gnarled hands reaching for the bottles. It was my mother's hands. Then they showed a car door opening and these legs trying to get out with a cane. And it was just the damnedest experience. It was very strange to be a viewer to a piece of your own life, poked right in front of you on the TV screen with no warning. I can still see that living room and the way the light of day was."

Karla's efforts to get the media involved had spread beyond the Halifax area. Television reporter Susan Ormiston's item on the old lady with AIDS who had been denied entry into nursing homes struck a chord and was carried widely in Canada.

Nursing home operators and provincial government ministers made excuses why this elderly woman was being denied. Lloyd Brown, president of Northwood, spoke of the fear staff and residents at the home would have of being in daily contact with an AIDS patient in the laundry or dining rooms.

"What's important here is how people feel about it, not the realities," Brown told Ormiston on camera. He mentioned the paranoia that hit Nova Scotia over another AIDS case involving a teacher. And he told other journalists that Northwood just did not have an action plan to deal with AIDS patients. Admitting Eva would just worsen the situation, he argued.

Tom McInnis, then provincial community services minister, was pressed by the media for action. The government cannot force nursing homes to take a patient, he replied. Members of the public are afraid they will contract the disease. "You have a public outcry, a fear of the unknown."

Karla had been told that if she went public she would be fired from Northwood. But she had another card to play. After what she describes as "an incredibly bad week," Karla had her mother admitted again to the Victoria General Hospital. "Once I got her in, I told her what I planned to do — refuse to take her home." At first her mother was hysterical, but Karla was adamant. "I told her you can be a miserable bitch or you can join me in this fight, but I'm going to do it. Then she came around to my side."

Karla told the hospital staff she would not take her mother home any more. A place would have to be found for her. They told her it would cost $536 a day to keep her mother in the hospital. Karla told Eva to phone Susan Ormiston if they closed down her bed. And if she was sent any bills, they should go to Susan as well.

This was not as hard-hearted as it sounds. Each day, Karla would drive up to the hospital in a jeep, a nurse would help Eva aboard, and mother and daughter would spend time together until it was time to return for the night. But the tactic paid off.

Northwood came up with an independent apartment for Eva for about six months, until she got sick and no one would take care of her. Karla renewed her game playing until finally a bed was found.

Karla says Eva had a wonderful will to fight, but then one day she decided it was enough. "In the last couple of weeks, she said, 'Have I won everything I can win?' And she said, 'Next summer, you're not going to live without your husband.'"

Eva Blaikie died July 4, 1989. She is buried in her home village of Upper Stewiacke, Nova Scotia.

Today, Karla does AIDS volunteer work in the small New Brunswick town where she lives with her family. She says that smaller communities have special trouble coping with AIDS. "They are still very backward," she muses. "That part is very sad." Some people are still afraid to talk about AIDS. "One day they will."

Even now, five years after Eva's death, the Blaikie family had reservations about going public. This book is the first time they have been willing to tell their story and be identified.

In the end, Northwood produced a manual on how to handle patients with AIDS. It was dedicated "To Eva Blaikie and her daughter Karla." The dedication was written by Lloyd Brown, whom they had to fight to get Eva admitted into the home.

"He was changed by what happened," Karla says simply.

Chapter 14

BAD BLOOD, PART TWO

"It is unfortunate that there are misconceptions that only
HIV infection has catastrophic effects."
DR. MAN-CHIU POON, FORMER CHAIR OF THE CANADIAN HEMOPHILIA
SOCIETY'S MEDICAL ADVISORY COMMITTEE, MAY 1991

Etienne Saumure's persistence finally got results. Saumure is a Gatineau, Quebec, hemophiliac who dodged the HIV bullet but was stricken by another virus carried in the blood, hepatitis C (also known as HCV). As liver disease progresses, the grey-haired man in his early fifties has become increasingly ill and beset by depression. His wife, Lise, has also been infected.

With all the focus on AIDS, little attention had initially been paid to this strange breed of hepatitis, even though people infected with HIV through use of blood are also very likely to be hit by hepatitis C. In most cases, the impact of HCV is not as dramatic as HIV. Saumure himself had lost a hemophiliac brother to AIDS. But in a minority of infections, like Saumure's, hepatitis C can be severely debilitating.

Saumure, faced with the heavy cost of drugs to fight his disease and an inability to work, wondered aloud in public why his infection should not be covered by government assistance. It came through blood, ultimately may kill its victims, and in at least some cases might have been prevented by the use of a surrogate test. He complains that he, too, was administered bad blood, but he got the wrong disease.

When the Krever inquiry was established, there was finally an opportunity to put hepatitis C infection on the public agenda.

Saumure seized the moment and engaged a lawyer, Pierre Lavigne, who doggedly raised the subject throughout the hearings. For this, Saumure deserves credit. The Hemophilia Society, preoccupied with HIV infections, is now paying more attention to HCV. And a national HCV-infected, blood-transfused group started in Toronto and has spread across much of Canada.

HIV is only one of more than a score of viruses known to be transmitted through blood. Before HIV came along, a variety of liver-damaging hepatitis viruses were feared by blood-products users. In fact, the earliest heat-treated products were preparations designed to kill hepatitis B, and they were not always terribly successful. Some of those who escaped HIV infection, ironically, had chosen the treatment that saved them because they were trying to avoid hepatitis.

There was another hepatitis virus lurking in the blood system before the AIDS epidemic. Researchers had been unable to pin it down, but they knew it was something different than those previously identified. They called it, for want of a better name, non-A, non-B hepatitis, shortened to NANB. As further discoveries were made, it was found NANB was actually a number of viruses, the most common of which was labelled hepatitis C.

As if one burden wasn't enough, it was found that many HIV-infected blood-products users were also hit by HCV. But that isn't all. Today we know that HCV infection through blood is actually very much more common than HIV, and that thousands of cases might have been prevented by use of tests available in 1986.

Hepatitis C is of a different family of viruses from the others identified and labelled as A, B, D, and E. The virus, which may be related to yellow fever, was isolated and cloned in 1989.

With the attention directed at HIV contamination because of imminent and frequent deaths among tainted blood victims, the problem of hepatitis C has largely been overlooked until now. Yet hundreds of people in Canada may have been infected every year.

Victims of this infection are still turning up. Some hemophiliacs, for example, didn't find out they were HCV-positive until late 1993 when a modern generation of more sensitive tests was introduced. It's almost certain their infection occurred some years ago, before the viruses were eliminated in the newer breed of blood products, according to medical authorities.

Dr. Tom Bowen of Calgary, a former Red Cross medical director, pointed out the difference in attitude towards the two viral diseases when he appeared before the Krever inquiry. Hepatitis NANB was around twenty years before AIDS, he said, and it was not brought under control because no one took on extraordinary measures — a hit list — to isolate the virus.

There remain many unanswered questions about HCV. It seems eerily reminiscent of the HIV virus a decade ago, striking hardest at some of the same populations that are vulnerable to AIDS. Sharing of contaminated needles, as well as blood transfusions, are among the chief means of transmission. Heart-surgery patients and victims of the disease thalassemia are also vulnerable. But a large proportion of HCV-infected persons — perhaps as high as 40 per cent — have no apparent history of exposure to the virus. There has been debate over the usefulness of a surrogate test, and people are still being notified they have the virus even though screening for HCV itself was implemented in Canada in 1990. The Hemophilia Society was complaining as late as October 1994 that patients have not yet been informed of the results of HCV testing done several years ago. Some victims and families argue Canada should have followed the American lead and implemented surrogate testing in 1986. They denounce the delay as yet another failure of the national blood system.

If the federal Health Department's reaction is any indication, they have a point. The hands-off approach is very similar to the AIDS fiasco. A spokesman for the Bureau of Biologics was quoted in May 1994 as saying there is no point to try to trace recipients of HCV-infected blood. Doug Kennedy of the Bureau said there would be few public health benefits because there is "no vaccine or preventable treatment available." Ah, but there is drug therapy, Mr. Kennedy.

"The government has once again said: 'In the absence of anybody to take responsibility in providing medical help, we're going to leave a vacuum,'" one parent of two hemophiliac boys says bitterly.

As with AIDS, for most sufferers there is a latency period before the disease has a significant impact on the body. There's not much certainty how long that latent period lasts. Some doctors believe it could be as long as thirty years. Current estimates suggest only 10 per cent of HCV-infected persons will experience serious liver damage. HIV-positive people recall bitterly that was the same percentage some doctors suggested would progress to AIDS.

Other studies are more disturbing, suggesting a large proportion of chronic sufferers face serious risk of fatal liver disease some years down the road. A British survey indicated between 20 and 40 per cent of chronic patients will develop cirrhosis and predicted liver cancer in up to 15 per cent of patients. Most patients would not even show symptoms of the disease until cirrhosis is well advanced, the British researchers predict.

Some American estimates suggest that one in every two hundred multi-transfused persons, including hemophiliacs, will develop cirrhosis of the liver. The risk of infection with HCV through blood has now gone from about 10 per cent a few years ago, to about 0.2 per cent, some medical experts say.

Among vulnerable blood-users, rates of HCV infection vary, depending upon the severity and variety of the hemophilia or other disease, the kinds of blood products used, and the age of the victim. Some estimates suggest the HCV infection rate among severe hemophiliacs above the age of seven who used clotting concentrates before vapour heat treatment is close to 100 per cent. An estimated 70 per cent of all severe Canadian Factor VIII hemophiliacs are antibody-positive to hepatitis C, and the level is even higher, above 80 per cent, with severe Factor IX hemophiliacs. Another report says the rate among HIV-positive hemophiliacs is 77 per cent. This is akin to kicking someone when they are down. Studies suggest that HIV contributes to the faster replication of HCV, meaning quicker progression to liver failure.

The jury seems to be out on the frequency of infection by sexual contact, but physicians do suggest precautions be taken. At least one study has indicated that people with a large number of sexual partners are more likely to be at risk. And doctors have recommended that those infected should reduce their number of sexual partners and protect them against coming in contact with semen, vaginal secretions, saliva, and blood. One European study of forty-seven couples in which the male partner was an HCV-positive hemophiliac found no cases of infection in the women despite an average twelve years of unprotected sex. Conversely, an American study says sexual transmission might account for 6 per cent of cases. The Red Cross defers donors, at least temporarily, who have had sexual contact with persons with jaundice or hepatitis.

The vast majority of those infected with HCV through transfusion are believed to have been exposed before the introduction in the mid- to late 1980s of the blood products that underwent heat and solvent treatment to destroy lipid-coated viruses. Pooled clotting concentrates were believed to be a source, but HCV may have infected many people even before those products arrived, through use of cryoprecipitate or plasma.

But this doesn't tell the whole story. Canadian Red Cross estimates are that an average 0.074 per cent of blood donations tested in the early 1990s are positive to HCV. That's over twice as high a rate as hepatitis B and nearly 25 times higher than HIV during that time. Justice Krever, in his interim report on the blood system, says 648 donations were confirmed positive 1993. And some of this virus may still be slipping through the system. Screening tests now used in Canada miss 5 per cent of HCV-positive donations. Despite a range of cleansing methods like vapour heat, super-dry heat, and solvent-detergent treatments of blood-clotting concentrates, it's estimated that 2 per cent of hemophiliacs under age five have been infected. In

Canada, some doctors have warned ominously that HCV will in future be a significant cause of death among hemophiliacs. By mid-1994, liver damage caused by hepatitis C had been fatal to at least twelve hemophiliacs and two others had required risky liver transplants.

It's believed the global rate of HCV is considerably higher than that of HIV. That's not overly surprising, since hepatitis viruses have proven themselves to be harder to kill. Some estimates are that a half billion persons worldwide have the virus. In Canada, the infection rate is believed to be 0.52 per cent, meaning more than 140,000 persons have been hit. In the United States, the national rate is 1 per cent. An estimated one-third of Americans with chronic liver disease — that's inflammation of the liver longer than six months — are thought to have developed their condition through HCV. Liver cancer rates are still uncertain because of the latency period.

In July 1993, at a Congressional hearing in Washington, Jay Epstein, acting director of the Office of Blood Research and Review of the Food and Drug Administration, pointed out that the risk of hepatitis C infection in the United States is now "less than one in 3,300 per unit exposure." Epstein was pointing out the risk has dropped sharply, but he told the House of Representatives Oversight and Investigations sub-committee that the recent infection rate in transfusion recipients "translates into fewer than 5,400 cases of hepatitis C per year in the United States."

If the traditional rule of thumb that Canada is about one-tenth of the United States applies, it could mean up to 540 Canadians annually will be infected. An Ottawa specialist told a meeting of hemophiliacs in early 1994 that the infection rate in the United States "perhaps" translates into Canada. "It's a hot political question," she said.

If there's an optimistic note, it may be that the existing evidence suggests that HCV is not as deadly as HIV. According to the Canadian Liver Foundation, 50 per cent of people will have a mild, short-lived illness and clear the virus completely. Perhaps one in five persons will develop cirrhosis, or scarring, of the liver in a few years but in a majority of cases this vital organ will remain functional. Most people will not suffer from "significant disease." But a pamphlet published in August 1993 and written by Dr. Linda Scully of Ottawa adds a cautionary note: "Our knowledge of HCV infection is still in its early stages." Other medical authorities argue the results of HCV infection are more serious than previously thought, with recent evidence suggesting there is liver damage in up to four in every five cases of infection.

The disease has a number of effects. Swelling of the abdomen and ankles is common, varicose veins may develop in the esophagus and stomach with danger of rupture and severe bleeding, and there may be mental confusion when the liver is unable to cope with clearing the blood of accumulating poisons.

A minority of people who acquire HCV suffer severe effects soon after they are infected. One victim is Alan Powell, a Toronto man in his mid-fifties who underwent heart bypass surgery in 1986.

Powell describes himself as an advocate sociologist, a former professor at the University of Toronto who became a community consultant to citizens' groups. Founding chairman of Toronto's successful Stop Spadina Expressway committee, he has discovered a new cause — setting up a national organization known as the Canadian Association of Transfused Hepatitis C Survivors.

Once an active restaurant owner and media commentator, as well as being involved in his teaching and community activities, Powell found his health declining in the mid-1980s. He was in for a shock after the heart surgery that was supposed to give him a new lease on life. A month after his surgery he couldn't understand why he wasn't feeling any better. He had lost his appetite. "Then all of a sudden I turned yellow, first my eyes, and then I was yellow all over." Powell's memory suffered, his energy was sapped, and he was developing serious cirrhosis of the liver. He was very ill for about eighteen months.

"One of the consequences of serious hepatitis and serious liver disease is something called hepatic encephalopathy, the liver not being able to handle nutrients in the blood, turning them into ammonia, which floods the brain and you get very confused. I suffered through a lot of that then."

He raised questions with his doctors. "I'm not as sharp as I used to be," he complained. "I'm really stupid, I can't argue, I'm not on the ball."

They told him he was just getting old. "I said, 'There's something else going on here.' My cardiologist, a very dear man, said, 'You need a priest, not a doctor.'"

Powell was offered treatment with the then-experimental drug Interferon alfa-2b in 1988. Interferons are natural proteins produced by cells that have been invaded by a virus, which block the virus from multiplying. He was reluctant to have anything else intrude on his body, but agreed to consider it. Then they told him that after six months of treatment, they would have to do a liver biopsy.

"What does a biopsy entail and what are the risks?" he asked. One of the risks was a "one in a thousand" chance something could go wrong, there would be internal bleeding and he would require transfusions.

"I will do it providing I can have my own blood standing by. Autologous blood," he said. That wasn't possible, he was told.

"Well, I don't want any monkeying about my body any more," Powell replied. "I don't trust the blood system. I want nothing to do with someone else's blood."

Despite his early feelings about the drug test and the biopsy, he is now participating in a trial with another drug known as consensus interferon. He had to have a liver biopsy in June 1993 before starting the program, and that is when he found he had severe cirrhosis. When Powell was interviewed, he was pleased that one of his liver functions was down to normal for the first time since 1986, but he was also worried about fatigue, depression, and body aches.

Powell is angry at the Red Cross, believing that organization could have been screening blood for NANB hepatitis through surrogate tests even before HCV was identified. Had those tests been done in the early 1980s, he suggests, a large proportion of both HCV and HIV would have been eliminated from the blood supply. The cost would have been nothing compared with what those infections are now costing the health system.

He says he wants "an admission of guilt on an emotional level," money to help hepatitis C victims set up self-help groups to become educated, a system set up through which people can be quickly notified of disease, and "humane compensation" patterned after the Nova Scotia model to help people afford medication.

"I'm particularly worried about the cost of interferon," he says. The cost of up to $6,000 for a six-month course of treatment is not covered by provincial health plans and is especially punishing to victims with no private plans or those on welfare. "Four people in our group, in Toronto or Hamilton, are not taking the drug because they can't afford it."

In the fall of 1992, a national medical conference was held on HCV. Dr. Jerome Teitel, director of the adult hemophilia clinic at Toronto's St. Michael's Hospital, wrote in a report on the conference that the virus causes chronic hepatitis in a majority of cases.

"Most people do not become obviously ill with HCV, and the infection can only be detected by fluctuating abnormalities in blood tests of liver function," he wrote in an article printed in Hemophilia Ontario's spring newsletter in 1993. But some, he added, will ultimately develop long-term liver damage. "In some cases this can take the form of severe liver failure (cirrhosis) and possible liver cancer in a small proportion of people." Eventually, some HCV-infected people will require liver transplants when nothing more can be done for them, a scary prospect for persons with bleeding disorders. If your liver goes kaput and you also suffer from HIV, however, transplants are generally ruled out as an option.

Teitel said all blood donations used to produce Factor VIII and Factor IX are screened for HCV, and existing products are now treated to destroy the virus which may have escaped the safety net. "The risk of continued or new exposure to HCV via factor concentrates is now remote," he wrote.

Unlike hepatitis B, there is no vaccine for hepatitis C, but Interferon alfa-2b has been found effective in reducing inflammation and liver damage in many patients by eliminating the virus in 25 to 30 per cent of cases. Another one in four patients treated with injections of the drug show some early benefits but will have relapses when the initial six-month course of treatment is complete. They respond when given a second treatment. But interferon also causes side-effects in some patients — mood swings, irritability, depression, insomnia, nausea, and flu-like symptoms are among them. These are, unfortunately, much like the symptoms of the disease itself. Current treatment consists of interferon injections three times a week for six months. Some fortunate patients appear to clear the disease on their own. Still, the Hemophilia Society is pushing for interferon use immediately through drug trials, at no cost to people with HCV. Most hemophiliacs cannot qualify for drug insurance.

A disturbing feature to many people who are both HIV-positive and HCV-positive is that many of the drugs meant to protect the immune system or to combat opportunistic infections may have side-effects on the liver or other organs. AZT, the drug that some regard as the only effective drug against HIV itself, is one; Septra, taken to ward off *Pneumonocystis carinii* pneumonia, is another that can have harmful effects if the drug is not ingested with enough fluids. Despite that, the anti-AIDS drugs should be taken, says one doctor who treats scores of AIDS patients. If the choice is between death in fifteen months or death fifteen years down the road, you take your chances.

Unfortunately, HIV-positive patients also infected with HCV don't have a suitable drug that will fight off the progressive effects of both diseases. HIV-positive patients respond poorly to interferon — it can make them sicker. Persons with HIV are excluded, for instance, from the consensus interferon trial that Alan Powell is involved in, and the American FDA has not approved alfa-interferon for patients who carry both viruses.

The Red Cross has been evaluating a hepatitis C lookback program to see if it would be cost-effective to try to track down people exposed to hepatitis C that way. Some doctors suggest the best, and least costly, way of identifying transfusion patients who have been exposed is for those who are worried to have a test done on their own. They argue that many HCV-infected people will never show symptoms of any kind.

Medical economics enters the picture again. Surrogate testing of donations was being used in several countries, notably the United States, as early as 1986. Indeed, it had been recommended a couple of years before that by some American scientists who found a combination of two tests would pick up 61 per cent of NANB-positive blood units. After the virus was identified in 1989, testing for it began in Canada the following year. That specific identifier is now routinely used by the Red Cross to screen blood, with infected donations being removed from the system. But Canada never adopted the surrogate test. This decision ignited an international debate over whether surrogate testing was effective in reducing the spread of hepatitis C infection, or whether it was donor screening and heat treatment of blood products that has reduced the threat. The question is, if HCV had not been identified relatively quickly, would Canada still be fumbling about indecisively now?

In the late eighties, Canada lagged behind its neighbour in responding to the hepatitis C threat. The Americans, including blood-bankers chastened by the earlier debacle with HIV, recognized what a new round of infections could mean for them and began using surrogate tests in October 1986. The proposed testing combined hepatitis B core antigen and an enzyme known as alanine aminotransferase, or ALT. Levels of the enzyme rise in blood if there is liver damage and can be used as an "indirect marker of potential liver involvement," a Red Cross medical director told the Krever inquiry in 1994. There were drawbacks — a weekend drinking spree can set ALT levels rising in Monday-morning donations, and even obesity causes higher levels.

Canadian decision-makers dithered for four years after surrogate testing was widely introduced in the United States. The issue arose in Canada as early as June 1986 when an advisory sub-group to the Canadian Blood Committee discussed whether a surrogate test for non-A, non-B hepatitis would be scientifically valid. Debate had already begun in the United States, and the subject was placed on the agenda at the request of Roger Perrault of the Red Cross. In what appears to be a stunning degree of insensitivity, Perrault suggested that AIDS testing might be a fine surrogate for NANB.

"A discussion followed on ALT testing being carried out in the United States and the possible media and market pressure that could be placed on Canada to adopt this testing," read the meeting's minutes. "Dr. Perrault [then Red Cross national director for the blood transfusion service] warned that if the Red Cross were to adopt this testing, the cost could easily total $10 million." No decision was taken.

The issue was raised again in the advisory meetings in October 1987, fifteen months later. Dr. Gerry Growe, a hematologist and director of the hemophilia clinic at the Vancouver General Hospital, broached the subject a year after the introduction of surrogate testing in the United States. He noted the consensus between the American Association of Blood Banks and the National Institutes of Health that testing for ALT and hepatitis B core antibodies would be effective in reducing NANB hepatitis "significantly."

Dr. Brian McSheffrey, the Red Cross representative, was not impressed. The Red Cross was mulling over the possibility of doing a study in a few of its blood centres to obtain more recent information. McSheffrey indicated the Red Cross would rather the study proceed than implement testing.

Growe was incensed at the "sluggish response" to surrogate testing. "This is a travesty," he wrote in a letter to the Red Cross's British Columbia medical director. There was no reason to think Canadians would escape hepatitis C any more than people in the United States and in Britain, where surrogate testing was also being done.

In October 1988, it was reported the surrogate study had not yet begun at McMaster University. The cost of studying between 2,400 and 3,200 subjects was estimated at $2 million and there were difficulties locating funds and implementing the research. There was also the ethical question of how patient consent should be obtained. The Red Cross had suggested "the informed consent need not be obtained until *after* [their emphasis] the patients are transfused and that the consent itself be related only to the need for follow-up." The minutes of the meeting remarked: "The Ethics Committee of McMaster University has approved post-transfusion informed consent although this does not strictly adhere to the Medical Research Council guidelines." The discussion concluded with the necessity of a further meeting with National Health Research and Development Program referees to "discuss the propriety of 'bending' MRC guidelines with regard to informed consent." Eventually, the study subjects were asked to give "written informed consent."

By November 1989, the study was not even mentioned at an advisory meeting and NANB hepatitis infection was reported to be dropping, "probably a result of enhanced donor screening." Perrault said the Red Cross would recommend the implementation of direct HCV testing of donors as soon as test kits were available.

The study was proceeding at thirteen hospitals in Winnipeg, Hamilton, and Toronto when debate over surrogate testing took on an international dimension. A report in the *New England Journal of Medicine* in August 1992 suggested that before screening for surrogates, the risk in the United States of post-transfusion HCV was 3.8 per cent. The surrogate test reduced this infection risk to 1.5 per cent, and when the test for the virus itself was introduced, the risk dropped to 0.6 per cent, said American researcher Dr. James Donahue of Johns Hopkins University, and his colleagues.

A Canadian team led by Dr. Morris Blajchman of Chedoke-McMaster Hospital in Hamilton, then pursuing what was now called the post-transfusion hepatitis prevention project, questioned that this reduction was in fact due to surrogate testing. They noted the decline had occurred at a time when donors were being screened for HIV and heat treatment was being introduced. A letter to the *New England Journal* in April 1993 from Blajchman and two colleagues from

Toronto's Mount Sinai Hospital noted that the post-transfusion HCV infection rate in Canada in 1985 was 9.2 per cent. In the late 1980s, they said, that rate was less than 1.5 per cent. Since surrogate testing on blood donors had not been done in Canada, the improvement had to be due to improved donor screening, they argued.

Donahue and his co-workers stood firm. "Our data show an abrupt decrease in the rate of post-transfusion HCV when surrogate testing was introduced in October 1986," concluded Donahue. There was no further change in the rate of infection until May 1990 when the Red Cross implemented the actual test for the virus itself. Several countries that rejected surrogate testing, including Canada, Japan, and Spain, had higher post-transfusion infection rates than the United States in the years 1986 to 1989. Donahue noted that another Canadian study done in 1988 had pointed out the Canadian rate of post-transfusion HCV infection in 1985 and 1986 was twice as high as that of the United States. Of course, it's also possible that the higher rates of HCV infection in Canada which Donahue pointed out in the late 1980s occurred because donor screening and heat-treated blood products were introduced later in this country than south of the border.

Dr. Maung Aye, the Red Cross national director of blood services, defended the decision not to proceed with surrogate testing in a June 1994 interview. There was much debate in the United States, too, over the effectiveness of the tests, he noted. "Because of the confusion at the time, we decided to do a proper study to determine if surrogate testing was useful," says Aye. That work had taken years and found the tests did not add any degree of safety, he argued.

"When you are operating in a grey area, you can always err on the extreme safety side regardless of cost, and one day you'll be right, one day you'll be wrong. The Americans decided to do it. We didn't because we didn't have enough proof."

The Canadian Hemophilia Society forced the still-secret $3-million study into the open in the fall of 1994, obtaining a summary through Access to Information and making it public, an act that drew the wrath of Justice Horace Krever. The study's findings are contrary to the Red Cross interpretation expressed by Dr. Aye, and also compelled Blajchman to reverse his opinion.

Between 1988 and 1992, about 4,600 patients were divided into two groups and checked later for post-transfusion hepatitis. About half the patients received blood from a supply in which surrogate-positive units were removed, and the others got blood in which the surrogate-positive units were not withheld. Those who received the blood supply from which surrogate-positive units were not withheld were four times more likely, before the introduction of the HCV-antibody test in May 1990, to suffer from post-transfusion hepatitis. After the introduction of the HCV-antibody test, there was little difference between the two groups.

The surrogate test, the researchers concluded, "might have been of value" in reducing HCV infection before the antibody screening had begun. The body of the report was less tentative: The estimated benefit of NANB surrogate testing for post-transfusion HCV was 85 per cent before the antibody test for the virus was implemented. In fact, none of the first four hundred patients to receive the surrogate-screened blood got HCV. Five of the first four hundred to receive the unscreened blood did.

Blajchman acknowledged after his study was made public that intervention could have come sooner to stop infections by HCV. "Now that we know that the surrogate tests were of value, I have to say they would have been valuable to do way back when," he responded.

When the Hemophilia Society estimated that up to 12,000 Canadians may have been infected with hepatitis C because Canada did not follow the American lead on surrogate testing in 1986, that figure was not disputed.

In a brazen use of doublespeak, the report said: "The decision to introduce the NANB surrogate markers to screen blood donors in the United States was made without the benefit of data from prospective intervention studies showing efficacy." The "benefit" for Canadian transfusion recipients arising from the collection of that wonderful data seems to have been a higher hepatitis infection rate than their American counterparts.

What is significant for large numbers of HCV-infected victims is that surrogate tests might have red-flagged them several years earlier. They might have adopted a healthier lifestyle or started drug therapy. The risk of serious damage from hepatitis C can be compounded with delayed treatment and the continued consumption of liver-damaging alcohol. If you were infected by HCV in 1983 and only found out last year, that's more than a decade lost to therapy, or at least to a more appropriate lifestyle, both of which might check the adverse impact on the liver. Furthermore, some physicians say that if HCV infection is proven or presumed for ten years, patients must be considered for annual screening for liver cancer.

The fact is that for a span of several years, surrogate testing was one of the few cards available to play against the spread of hepatitis C. As in the case of HIV, the decision-makers opted to wait for absolute proof. And when a study funded by the Red Cross and federal government showed that decision to have been wrong, the information was withheld from the public. If a direct test for the virus hadn't been identified in 1990, Canadians might still be waiting for the guardians of their health to err on the side of safety.

Dr. Man-Chiu Poon, chair of the medical and scientific advisory committee to the Canadian Hemophilia Society, heard disturbing news early in 1991. Word had reached the Calgary-based doctor that the federal Health Department wanted plasma that carried hepatitis C antibodies returned to the pool that was used to manufacture a product known as immunoglobulin. He checked with Stephen Vick, responsible for manufacturing practices at the Red Cross, who not only confirmed that but told him the same plasma pool would be used to manufacture Factor VIII clotting concentrates. More confirmation came in a letter dated February 19, 1991, by Dr. Susan Robinson of Halifax, chair of the MSAC's blood products sub-committee.

Immediately, Poon wrote to the head of the Bureau of Biologics, to oppose the pooling of HCV-positive plasma. The policy should be re-examined and the ruling retracted, he said. Although the products made from the plasma would be treated to kill viruses, the viral inactivation of concentrates is "by no means perfect," the doctor pointed out.

A month later he received a reply from Dr. Wark Boucher, acting director of the Bureau. Boucher said he was not aware of any ruling that HCV-positive plasma could be returned to the pools. Only screened plasma could be used to produce coagulation products, he said. On the other hand, Boucher added, there was overwhelming evidence that immunoglobulin produced from plasma unscreened for hepatitis C was safe and changes in manufacturing practices were not justified. In a later note, he added "this did not mean that only non-reactive plasma should be used for (coagulation) products."

Poon replied to Boucher in May 1991 with the "sad reminder that at least seven Canadians had been infected with HIV by Factor VIII concentrates subjected to a viral inactivation procedure then approved by the Bureau of Biologics." He mentioned this had led to legal action being taken. The use of unscreened plasma or plasma supplemented with HCV-positive plasma "will invite disaster," Poon said. "There is no room for complacency in the foreseeable future." Intentional or unintentional bypass of safety procedures is a breach or safe practice and is not responsible, Poon complained. "It is unfortunate that there are misconceptions that only HIV infection has catastrophic effects."

Poon said he was pleased the Red Cross was only using non-HCV-reactive plasma for Canadian blood-clotting concentrates and said he expected the practice would continue. "We also expected the Bureau of Biologics to require all coagulation factor concentrates for use by Canadian patients at all times be manufactured only from HCV-screened non-reactive source plasma irrespective of the countries of origin of the source plasma and the location of the manufacturers."

Response from the federal government was slow. Poon wrote twice more in 1991, the second time in October backed by motions from the MSAC and the hemophilia clinic directors. He noted that the American Food and Drug Administration had reversed an earlier decision that had been imitated in Canada and had now fallen in line with other "developed" European countries and Australia. "There is no reason why Canada, as a leader in health care, should procrastinate further," he said in one letter. "Hepatitis C infection causes significant morbidity," Poon added, noting it was linked to hepatocellular carcinomas (liver cancer) as a long-term health hazard.

It wasn't until November 15, 1991, that Dr. J. Furesz, the Bureau's director, issued an order to all manufacturers of blood products that effective January 1, 1993, all human plasma for the production of those blood products used in Canada — no matter the country of origin — shall be screened for antibodies to HCV using an approved test. Furthermore, the Bureau assured Poon later, all Canadian-source plasma would be screened for HCV antibodies. The federal regulator, which has a duty to protect Canadians from hazardous biological products, had taken nine months to act.

Poon also had another target. The Factor IX concentrate for hemophilia B patients that was favoured by the Red Cross, for contractual reasons, was AlphaNine, a high-purity product made by the California-based firm Alpha Therapeutics. He was concerned that some researchers had found traces of HCV in the product and that the virus-killing process used might not be completely effective.

In May 1991, Poon wrote Alpha saying that unless he could be assured that HCV was not a problem in Alpha High Purity products, he could not recommend their use. He wanted an assessment of random lots done by independent labs. Poon also warned his colleagues treating hemophilia B patients: "Until you are certain that the Alpha High Purity Factor IX will not transmit HCV, you may not want to use it for certain patients." Mild cases and patients who were now HCV-negative, especially, should avoid the product.

If it were not for Poon's determined initiative, it's possible even more blood users would have been infected with hepatitis C.

Could hepatitis C develop into a life-threatening pandemic, like AIDS? We don't know at this stage. Information about the impact of this virus is still scant, but recent evidence suggests liver damage is likely in up to 80 per cent of HCV-infected hemophiliacs, for example.

And who knows what other viruses could be lurking in the blood supply? "We're working our way through the alphabet," Red Cross medical director Dr. Roslyn Herst told the Krever inquiry in February 1994. That expanding alphabet soup was one reason many doctors embraced a new generation of purer, cleaner plasma-derived and synthetic products in 1993.

Chapter 15

THE FIGHT FOR SAFETY

"It's exactly the same inefficient system we had ten years ago
when so many Canadians were infected with the AIDS virus."
TOM ALLOWAY, PRESIDENT OF HEMOPHILIA ONTARIO, NOVEMBER 1993

Canada's blood bureaucrats should have been mortified at the first
public hearing in November 1993 of Justice Horace Krever's inquiry
into the tainted blood scandal.

Six weeks earlier, yet another wrinkle to the international bad
blood scandal had emerged in Germany. UB Plasma, a private firm,
had been selling plasma that was improperly tested for HIV to pharmaceutical companies in several European countries. The firm was
shut down and the management arrested. Later, a second German
company, Haemoplas, faced similar accusations. As the scandal
unfolded, Germany's health minister advised ten million of his com-
patriots who had received blood transfusions since 1980 to be tested
for the virus. The foul-up was called the most serious health crisis in
the history of Germany's federal republic.

No one should have been surprised that questions would be asked
about whether any products made from the suspect blood had found
their way to Canada. Early in November, the Canadian subsidiary of
Austrian-based Immuno AG announced the withdrawal of a preparation known as Immune Serum Globulin used to protect travellers
against hepatitis A, because the parent company had purchased blood
from UB Plasma. Assurances were given that there was nothing to

worry about. In withdrawing its product, Gammabulin, Immuno was just being extremely cautious and acting out of public concern. Anyway, Immuno said, the product had been heat-treated, so there was no danger.

Both the Red Cross and Health Department officials rushed to the barricades to assure users of clotting concentrates that there was no problem. Canada had not imported any potentially risky factors.

They were wrong, and spent the next three weeks scraping traces of egg from their faces.

The Canadian Hemophilia Society could not have orchestrated a more eye-catching debut to the Krever inquiry. When the German affair broke, Lindee David, the Society's executive director, and Durhane Wong-Rieger, then vice-president, pestered suppliers, regulators, and distributors to determine whether the assurances were correct. After two weeks, they were told that two lots of a heat-treated Factor IX concentrate made by Immuno from UB Plasma's material had imported into Canada and distributed by the Red Cross. The expiry dates of the lots had been September 1992 and March 1993, so by that time it was very likely the product had already been used, possibly by as many as two hundred Factor IX hemophiliacs. As a precaution, on November 22 the Red Cross called back any unused vials of the three million units imported into Canada.

Failure to communicate was stamped all over the affair. A Red Cross chronology says Immuno assured its officials on November 5 that there were no UB Plasma–source products distributed in Canada. On November 15, however, Immuno contacted the federal Bureau of Biologics about the two lots of Factor IX. Red Cross officials say they were not told by either the Bureau or Immuno.

Dr. Maung Aye, the Red Cross national director of blood services, says it was difficult obtaining information. "I was running from one magazine shop to another picking up all the German magazines and newspapers and having them translated overnight, because there was no other way of getting information. I called colleagues in Europe. After a while, I said, This is stupid, this is not the way to run a blood program." He decided to send a team to check out the manufacturer in Vienna.

Clinics and hospitals had been alerted, but even here there was confusion and attempts to downplay what was happening. One nurse told the mother of a Factor ix hemophiliac that the fuss over Immuno's product in Canada was "old news" and no one had been infected. That assessment was given at the same time that both the Red Cross and the federal Health Department had dispatched teams to beautiful Vienna to poke through Immuno's manufacturing records. If it was old news, the travelling investigators must have spent their visiting time in the Austrian capital, up to a week, enjoying Sachertorte by the less than blue Danube.

The bureaucrats felt sure any danger that may have lurked in blood supplied by UB Plasma had been overcome by heat processing. "All the records and documents were found to be in order and indicate that Immuno's production methods met excellent international standards," the Red Cross reported. "Health Canada is confident that all products are free of hiv," federal officials said on November 26.

The scare was over, but it was the Hemophilia Society staff and members who had recognized the potential implications. The debacle revealed there were still flaws in the system. They had pointed out that Immuno products which might have been contaminated had found their way through the maze. Furthermore, it was the consumer group, not the regulators, distributor, or funders who blew the whistle.

"It has taken three weeks of vigorous action on our part," chs president David Page told the opening day of the Krever inquiry. He added that while the product was not a risk, it showed there were problems. "We want to make sure it doesn't happen again."

Tom Alloway, Hemophilia Ontario's president, went further in a television interview. "This incident shows that we still do not have an effective emergency response mechanism," he said bitterly. "The Canadian Bureau of Biologics, the part of the federal government supposed to monitor safety of products, did not have an efficient way of responding to this. It's exactly the same inefficient system we had ten years ago when so many Canadians were infected with the AIDS virus."

"This was, in essence, an unplanned test of Canada's current ability to respond to a potential emergency in the blood system," wrote Wong-Rieger. The Society's medical advisory committee called the incident the first test of the safety alert activating mechanism of the Canadian blood system since 1986. Had the blood system been a student, it would have rated a D-minus.

One might think, with HIV and hepatitis victims as daily reminders, that those who control the blood supply would be extraordinarily cautious, using whatever means were at hand to prevent new dangers from occurring. Any new bug that creeps into the blood supply could put all consumers at additional risk. Problems would show up among the most blood-dependent group, the hemophiliacs, first.

Medical experts often point out that human blood is a potentially hazardous drug and can never be completely safe. "The safest blood is no blood," Dr. Annette Poon of Toronto's Hospital for Sick Children told the Krever inquiry. One hundred per cent safety is "not an achievable objective," said another hematologist, Dr. Peter Pinkerton of Toronto's Sunnybrook Hospital. It's common sense that purer is most likely to be safer.

But the best possible defence against unknown new viruses was apparently not a priority of some stakeholders in Canada's blood establishment in the early 1990s. For years, the dream of hemophiliacs and others who relied on blood was that safe, artificially produced products, free of viral contamination, could be made available. Properly made and carefully tested, these new products could end the risk of foreign infective agents in the blood. When they arrived, however, governments were reluctant to pay for them.

In the late 1980s, ultra-high-purity monoclonal and recombinant (synthetic) Factor VIII products were developed. Both represented major steps towards a truly safe blood supply for hemophiliacs. Recombinant, especially, offered a product free of the harmful viruses that had killed many hemophiliacs and the potential for a supply that would be available even if there were plasma shortages.

Monoclonal concentrate, although plasma-derived, is purified by Baxter of California via a process that passes cryoprecipitate through a column in which antibodies selectively extract Factor VIII. The product is also treated with a solvent detergent which dissolves the lipids, or fatty coatings, on viruses such as HIV, hepatitis B, and hepatitis C, thus wiping out those threats to people who need blood products. Finally, the product is freeze-dried. Baxter touts its Hemofil M as the most advanced concentrate made from plasma and promotes the company's hard-nosed donor screening as an extra protection against contamination. Hemofil M was actually licensed for use in Canada in 1988, but until 1993 was seldom used because the Canadian Blood Agency and its predecessor, the Canadian Blood Committee, would not pay for it.

Both monoclonal and recombinant products are not entirely "pure." Hemofil M and recombinant factors have small amounts of mouse or hamster cells added. In the case of Miles-Cutter's recombinant product Kogenate, the concentrate is produced from hamster kidney cells into which the human Factor VIII gene has been inserted. The product is purified further to remove potential contaminants. Severe hemophiliacs might hesitate briefly if challenged with the ancient question, Are you man or mouse?

Furthermore, because the concentration of the clotting factor is so high, human albumin is added to stabilize the Factor VIII. The good news is that albumin is a pasteurized protein that has an excellent safety record and no known impact on the immune system. If there was truth in advertising, a tongue-in-cheek Dr. Jerome Teitel told a 1994 Hemophilia Ontario meeting, the product description of the synthetic concentrate would be plasma-derived albumin contaminated by a little bit of recombinant Factor VIII.

These new factors are in a different league than the Koate-HP that was the mainstay for Canadian Factor VIII hemophiliacs during the late 1980s and early 1990s. Koate contains about 50 to 60 units of active factor per milligram. The monoclonal and recombinant concentrates have activity that ranges between 2,000 and 4,500 units. "It is important to remember that intermediate purity concentrates are, in fact, not terribly concentrated," American specialist Peter Levine wrote in a British newsletter. "They contain less than one per cent clotting factor concentrate and more than 99 per cent extraneous and unnecessary proteins from the many donors who have contributed to the pool. The new high-purity products, after purification by monoclonal antibody technology, are less than one per cent impurities and more than 99 per cent clotting factor, prior to the addition of albumin."

Despite the exceptionally high purity, there were concerns. In 1992, some doctors called for further testing of recombinant factor before its general introduction into Canada. No other country had gone after recombinant factors full-bore, although clinical trials had been conducted in Europe and the United States. While the new synthetics eliminated known viruses from the picture, no one could be sure what the long-term effects of infusing artificial recombinant products would be.

There was also some concern with monoclonal factors. While the solvent-detergent process used in monoclonal production would destroy lipid-enveloped viruses, plasma-derived concentrates would always be theoretically vulnerable to the appearance of new viruses.

Until the fall of 1993, these cleaner clotting factors — with a very few exceptions — were not available to Canadians. Despite the bitter and well-documented history of HIV and hepatitis, Canadian hemophiliacs have had to struggle against inert provincial governments and vested corporate interests to have safer products made available to them.

The bleak history of the last decade has left blood-product consumers nervous about the supply. A June 1993 survey of hemophiliacs, before the new products were available, found much concern about the risk of contracting new "unknown" viruses through infusions. There was also substantial fear that some AIDS virus might slip through the screening and viral inactivation process, concern over the sources of blood products, and anxiety about being treated by professionals who didn't know what they were doing. On the other hand, only 30 per cent of respondents thought they could get better blood products in other countries.

Meanwhile, the wheeling and dealing over the blood products seems to be off-limits to consumers. Hemophiliacs were not consulted when the five-year contract between the Red Cross and Cutter that initially went into effect in 1989 was extended by the parties until 1996. Details have been a guarded secret—"proprietary information." The Canadian Hemophilia Society has been denied access to the contract. It's believed the pact gives Cutter the right to process all Canadian plasma collected by the Red Cross and used to make clotting concentrates. In the fall of 1994, that point potentially threatened the production of plasma-derived factors for Canada. There was also a guarantee that allows the replacement of the older Cutter product if something better comes along.

When it came to costs, the Society — and even the governments that pay the bills — found the information was secret. When pressure grew for the switch to the new products, the old bugbear of money came up. The trouble is, the consumers were unable to find out the exact costs.

In December 1992, a breakthrough occurred at Canada's Health Department when federal authorities approved Baxter's Recombinate, the first synthetic product licensed for general use in Canada. That was followed in June 1993 by the licensing of Kogenate, Miles-Cutter's equivalent. This licensing did not have any immediate impact on Canada's hemophiliacs. The Canadian Blood Agency did not fund these new, more pricey concentrates for routine use, and it appeared the Agency was in no rush to alter its stance.

Ultra-high-purity products were already being used in several countries, promoted by doctors who believed that the unwanted protein clutter existing in standard plasma-derived products compromised the immune system. No one in Canada seriously questioned the safety of the previous breed of products, although there's always concern new dangers — such as Chagas disease, originating from Latin America — could appear in plasma-source material. But what pushed Canadian hemophiliacs towards the ultra-high-purity products were research findings in the United States and Western Europe of improved immune response in HIV victims within six months of discontinued use of the older, less pure products. It made sense — clean up all the extraneous junk from the concentrates and the body's immune system can spend its energy fighting more troublesome enemies. Furthermore, some doctors said use of recombinant Factor VIII would eliminate the danger of new hepatitis C cases. When the news was disseminated, pressure grew for a switch to the new concentrates.

In March 1993, hemophilia clinic directors met with the Red Cross and the Canadian Blood Agency and resolved that recombinant Factor VIII should be the treatment of choice for classical hemophilia. Previous concerns about recombinant factors had been addressed, they said.

The directors' recommendation for a switch to recombinant Factor VIII caught CHS officials off guard. The clinic directors' decision was at odds with the stance of the CHS, which wanted individual hemophiliacs to have a choice of available products.

Wong-Rieger, who took over the CHS presidency in May 1994, says what had driven the clinic directors' recommendations were the contracts the Red Cross has with existing suppliers. The old Miles-Cutter and Red Cross link, stronger than ever since the two corporations had put together a proposal for a Canadian blood fractionation plant in Nova Scotia, was one of the forces at work. Miles-Cutter, she says, had offered $1 million of free recombinant to physicians.

The Red Cross and Miles-Cutter romance has been one of the longest-lasting corporate relationships during these turbulent years in the blood industry. Overall, there's little denying the company has produced consistently good products. But even when Cutter's technology lagged behind its competitors, it seems to have been given preference by the Red Cross.

A supporter might argue that the reason for the preference is Cutter's consistency. A cynic might suggest it's because Cutter pays back 5 per cent of the contract value into a research and development fund for Red Cross researchers. That sweetheart arrangement dates back at least to the start of the contract between the Red Cross and Cutter, signed in 1989. (The deal, incidentally, was hailed by the Hemophilia Society at the time.) The Red Cross defends the clause, saying all bidders were asked to include an "R&D mechanism" in the contract bids they submitted.

When the Hemophilia Society started delving into the question of costs of the new products, a very uncompetitive scenario emerged.

Cutter made both Koate, the older product, and its recombinant Kogenate. It did not make a monoclonal concentrate. Eliminate Baxter's monoclonal from the picture and Cutter would have a virtual stranglehold on the Canadian Factor VIII market. The Red Cross also had a contract with the U.S. firm Alpha Therapeutics for Factor IX. This is the product that Dr. Man-Chiu Poon of Calgary, then chief medical advisor to the CHS, warned doctors against using in 1991 until there was proof it would not transmit hepatitis C. The CHS wanted a monoclonal product made by the Austrian firm Immuno to be available, too. The CHS was told it could be supplied with all the recombinant it wanted. But the Society held firm — it wanted monoclonal available to its members as well.

The Red Cross said the contract allowed them to bring in Cutter recombinant as a substitute for the old Koate, but would not allow substitution by monoclonal, made by Baxter. Indeed, they said, the use of monoclonal would mean a penalty and it would end up costing more than recombinant factor, even though the per-unit cost for the plasma-derived product was considerably less than that of Cutter's recombinant. Let's buy out the contract, get out of it, Wong-Rieger suggested.

We can't, she was told. Canada's Red Cross collection centres are not licensed by the U.S. Food and Drug Administration and only Cutter, which has a grandfather clause in their contract pre-dating the FDA requirement, could send Canadian plasma to the United States. A rival like Baxter would not be able to process Canadian plasma because the Red Cross did not meet FDA standards. The winter of 1993 was the first time the CHS learned that Canadian collection centres were not FDA-approved and that they must be FDA-licensed for plasma to be shipped to the United States.

Meanwhile, the Canadian Blood Agency argued that governments would not allow wholesale switching to the new, more expensive products because of increased costs and the trimming of health budgets. The agency wanted a phased-in introduction, with a set of priority consumers drawn up as was done during the heart-rending and distasteful process of 1985. The Society did a membership survey and found the majority wanted everyone to get the new products at the same time. Hemophiliacs refused to do the kind of ugly priorization that had occurred in 1985. They demanded a 100-per-cent switch-over.

As the cat-and-mouse games were being played, inquiries from individual hemophiliacs about the availability of the new products were being brushed off. A request made in the spring of 1993, through a hemophilia clinic director and the Red Cross, for either monoclonal high purity or recombinant Factor VIII for an HIV-infected hemophiliac was turned down. The products were not approved for funding by the CBA.

The Canadian Blood Agency was to meet in late May 1993 to decide whether the provinces would be willing to pay for the new products. David Page, then president of the Canadian Hemophilia Society, did not seem overly confident the bid would be approved. The cost of widespread use of the latest generation of products could be $50 million more.

In this fight, however, the CHS was not alone. Their medical and scientific advisory committee wanted action, and clinic directors across the country openly supported use of the recombinant concentrates. It would help, some grassroots hemophiliac families felt, if there was a sign that they wanted them, too.

My wife, Lorraine Calderwood-Parsons, thought a demonstration to reinforce the demand for the new products would get the message across. She received backing from the Ottawa regional board and from Hemophilia Ontario. An idea was to send a delegation to the CBA meeting to confront the provincial representatives face-to-face, to let them know what impact the decisions bureaucrats made would have on their lives. A letter-writing campaign was launched. Tom Alloway wrote Ontario Health Minister Ruth Grier pointing out that past "economy measures" were responsible for the AIDS catastrophe and also for the infection by hepatitis C of many patients with von Willebrand's disease.

William Dobson, executive director of the Agency, was nervous when Lorraine told him about the demonstration. He recognized there was a lot of anxiety and anger among hemophiliacs. "I don't want to be put in a situation where our representatives will be verbally abused. What we need is a certain level of calmness," said Dobson.

"We won't verbally abuse your members if you promise to stop physically abusing ours," Lorraine retorted.

The Canadian Hemophilia Society was making a formal pitch to the Agency and Page was afraid a protest might backfire. After some discussion, during which it was pointed out that the action would show grassroots support for national officers, Page agreed. Meanwhile, thousands of letters supporting the introduction of the new products were collected and sent to health ministers.

The demonstration was held May 26 in front of the Canadian Blood Agency headquarters in Ottawa. Some provincial representatives on the Agency, including the board member from Quebec, came and spoke informally to the seventy people who turned up. Besides Ottawa, hemophiliacs and supporters came from central Ontario, nearby Quebec, and even from British Columbia.

Montreal-area hemophiliacs declined to attend, apparently nervous that a protest would rankle provincial officials then involved in HIV-compensation talks.

A day later, a small representative group, led by Alloway, was invited into a half-hour meeting with the Agency directors. One of them was John Meyers, a hemophiliac with AIDS who died within months but was determined to leave his mark. Besides Alloway and Meyers, the group included the wife of an HIV-positive hemophiliac, a couple with a son who was not HIV-positive but who had been made ill by another blood-borne virus, and the fifteen-year-old sister of another HIV-positive hemophiliac. Some directors were moved to tears by the appeals.

On May 28, the Agency announced the approval of the phased introduction of monoclonal and recombinant Factor VIII and high-purity Factor IX. "The high purity level of these products lessens the threat of infection from viruses, and is also believed to play a part in stabilizing the immune system," a news release said. By the end of 1993, the majority of Canadian hemophiliacs were using the new products, and Canada is the first country to completely fund recombinant clotting factor. Other countries are watching the Canadian experience with interest.

By the spring of 1994, Canadian hemophiliacs outside Quebec were using 65 per cent recombinant factor, 10 per cent monoclonal, and 25 per cent had stuck with Koate. Quebec was just then adopting the new products. The purported reason for the delay in Quebec was that the province wanted to do a scientific evaluation, but Page says if a review was done, the government had not asked any of the hemophilia experts for their input. The delay in Quebec was more likely for budgetary reasons.

In June 1994, some HIV-positive Quebec hemophiliacs were rattled by a recommendation from their specialists that they stick with the intermediate product they had used for five years. The high-purity products were not worth the risk that inhibitors might develop, they were told. When inhibitors develop and are severe, the body will not tolerate the injection of foreign Factor VIII and the clotting concentrate does not work. The doctors argued that if hemophiliacs had been using the old product for years without inhibitors developing, they were likely safe from that threat.

David Page, who lives in the Quebec City area, says several doctors had told him that the last thing an HIV-positive hemophiliac needed was inhibitors. "They weren't convinced that the research showed any advantage to the higher purity products in terms of CD-4 counts and overall health, and they think there's a theoretical risk, at least, when you switch products," Page said in August 1994. "Research I saw in Mexico [at an AIDS conference] didn't seem to show any greater risk when you do the same kind of study with the same kind of people."

The doctors did not refuse to prescribe the new products, and admitted the high-purity concentrates were superior in stopping new viruses that might enter the blood supply. But they wanted patients to sign a document that they had been informed. "Given the context, with everybody blaming the doctors, they are being very careful," remarked Page.

An insert in boxes of Miles-Cutter's recombinant factor does mention the risk of "neutralizing antibodies," which appeared in about one-fifth of previously untreated hemophilia patients. But Page says inhibitors might have been discovered because researchers are looking harder than ever before. "When you look hard for anything, you'll find it. A lot of these inhibitors are at a fairly low level and disappear." Page also says costs may have concerned some Quebec doctors, "although they won't admit it." One specialist has made remarks to him like "You're working, so you're worth the huge cost of products."

It's also "more than a possibility," Page says, that stocks of the old product no longer in demand in the other provinces were shipped to Quebec for use there. "Nine of the ten provinces made their decision on the best guess about health and Quebec didn't go along with it. It seems strange that Quebec would have its own creature, the Canadian Blood Agency, and wouldn't go along with it for scientific reasons."

* * *

Did the tainted blood scandal of the 1980s make federal regulators pay more attention to the integrity of the blood system? This is one of the great shortcomings of the past, and present, blood systems. The ideal and the reality don't mesh. A former senior regulator in the Bureau of Biologics said in 1993 that "we generally will try to do an inspection every other year in a facility." That's looking at the inspection system with rose-coloured glasses.

Dann Michols, executive director of Health Canada's drugs directorate and the national pharmaceutical strategy, found himself in a bit of a corner before the Krever inquiry in February 1994. Michols, who had joined the Health Department two years before, said all Red Cross blood collection centres were inspected and licensed after blood was added to the Food and Drugs Act schedule of hazardous drugs in 1989. The policy was to try to inspect the centres every two years, Michols added. "We have since changed that to inspecting every year."

Krever asked if the policy had been followed.

"As resources would allow, yes," replied Michols tentatively.

Did resources allow each centre to be inspected every two years? Krever pursued.

"No. We inspected all of the centres the first year, 1989–90," Michols responded. "We will have inspected all of the centres this year, and we have dealt with priority cases of one type or another in the intervening period."

When asked by the inquiry lawyer Céline Lamontagne whether his answer meant there had been a lapse in inspections between 1990 and 1993, Michols fudged. "I am saying we did not inspect all of the centres within that two-year [sic] period. We have inspected all of the centres twice within the three-year period." Actually, the period Michols was referring to was a minimum of four years.

When an international expert, Dr. John Cash of Scotland's transfusion service, examined the Bureau in July 1994 on behalf of the Krever inquiry, he described the Agency's inspection of plasmapheresis operations as "remarkably sporadic and superficial." The audit of quality standards seems to have had a low priority in the Canadian blood system, he remarked. Red Cross staff had challenged the competence and authority of the inspectors. This eroded the morale of the Bureau and "encouraged them to avoid conflict by minimizing the frequency of visits and/or deliberately avoiding areas of perceived contention," Cash noted. It also led to a "cosy" relationship between the two groups. Federal regulators — the blood monitors — clearly suffered from low self-esteem.

Another foreign visitor, Dr. John Finlayson of the U.S. Center for Biologics Evaluation and Research, was equally critical after his tour in September 1994. "My general impression is of an organization that is vulnerable, if not utterly fragile," Finlayson wrote. A lack of staff and the inexperience of those who were there caught his eye.

From their recent hasty actions, federal authorities have admitted their inadequate role in the regulation of the blood system. Ottawa's bureaucrats may now recognize that they have had clear-cut regulatory authority and thus tremendous liability in the contaminated blood affair. Regulatory resources are being beefed up at a time when the prevailing order of the day is government cutbacks. Inspectors from the drugs directorate were trained to assist the four or five staff in the Bureau of Biologics who once carried out inspections. Furthermore, six new people were added to the previous twelve in the blood bank section in April 1993 and four more staff were to be hired in fiscal 1994–95. But is this enough? A report prepared for the Krever inquiry in November 1994, after those hirings were announced, stated the Bureau was "under-resourced" and the drugs directorate had not taken a leadership role.

Some believe the trouble with the Canadian regulatory system, at least as it applies to blood, has been lack of competence. "There has been no expertise in the system," complains one person who works in health regulation. Richard Huntsman, the Red Cross medical director in Newfoundland, told the Krever hearings that when inspectors arrived at his doors in the summer of 1994, they said they had never seen a hospital blood bank in operation or been in a public health laboratory. Krever says it is urgent that a competent inspection team be assembled.

Censored inspection sheets from the late 1980s and early '90s reveal a casual response by Red Cross regional centres to federal inspectors' criticisms. The centres would take from a year to twenty-one months to report on how problems were dealt with, although Huntsman says the paperwork lagged behind the remedies. Licences were renewed before problems were corrected.

In April 1989, for example, the Red Cross centre in London, Ontario, was criticized by a Bureau inspector for not having a clearly identified person responsible for quality control of blood. A year and a half later, the centre still had not established a quality assurance officer, a point noted in a second inspection.

The Saint John, New Brunswick, centre took sixteen months to reply to observations made by a regulator in July 1989. Months before the reply was sent back, the centre's licence expired, but a new one was issued before the problems identified had been addressed. That, an insider says, was routine.

In February 1986, a federal regulator demanded "immediate remedial action" to institute a program of tests of immunoglobulin at the Montreal centre. The same demand had been made in February 1984, but there had been no compliance.

The U.S. television program *Frontline* was told by a Food and Drug Administration regulator that when she objects to something, the inspected firm is very quick to show they have corrected the deficiency, or that they will do their best. Procrastinate and hope the problem disappears seems to have been the Canadian way.

The example of the centralized computer system, including a nationwide donor deferral registry linking the seventeen Red Cross collection centres, is a case in point. A condition of the licence issued to the Red Cross by the Bureau of Biologics in 1989 was that a computer system be set up. After several delays (one of six months because the CBA refused to hand over money), the $15 million system was to be up and running in early 1995, six years later.

Blood collected by the Red Cross for fractionation is now undergoing tougher scrutiny than ever before. Red Cross–collected plasma is shipped to a Miles-Cutter plant in North Carolina for processing into concentrates. Douglas Lindores, secretary-general of the Red Cross, admitted in early 1994 that Canadian blood collection centres would not pass American FDA inspections, which are the world's toughest. "It is essential to have FDA standards," Lindores told the Krever inquiry. Even if Canada was self-sufficient in blood products, it would still have to comply with the American FDA. "For legal reasons, we cannot fail to meet the highest world standard. If we didn't, we could theoretically be held negligent at some point for failing to adjust operations to take into account international standards."

It wasn't long before he was proven correct. In the summer of 1994, FDA inspectors started inspections of the seventeen Canadian Red Cross collection centres. They focused especially on plasmapheresis, or source plasma collection, in which the plasma is extracted from donors and the rest of their blood returned. Source plasma accounts for about a quarter of Canada's plasma supply. The Toronto centre was first under the gun, and the inspectors found nineteen violations of their standards. Some shortcomings were potentially serious — a failure to do tracebacks that identify all infected donors to a contaminated lot, incident reports that did not say how a problem was identified or that do not fully document investigations, or a lack of written follow-up on an estimated twenty-five to thirty mislabelled units per month. After the inspection, a truck that had been loaded with source plasma and was ready to leave for the United States was stopped. That happened on August 5, but the Red Cross kept the bad news to itself. It was a month before word of the failed inspection leaked out to the public.

By that time, other Red Cross centres had failed inspections. They were tumbling like dominoes. The centres had undergone

Bureau of Biologics checks earlier in the year and, while four had brief closures of their plasmapheresis operation, they had generally passed muster. Toronto's centre had thirty "observations" made by Bureau inspectors, but its operations never skipped a beat.

As news of the FDA inspection in Toronto surfaced, federal Health Minister Diane Marleau faced calls for her resignation. Damage control began. Lindores came forth and apologized for not making the reports public — that would be done in future, he pledged. And he admitted openly that there could be up to sixteen other failures, because all Red Cross collection centres now had to face two sets of rules from both the American and Canadian regulators. Marleau pledged to make efforts to "harmonize" the Canadian and American standards. "The systems are different," she said. "One is not necessarily better than the other." Lindores welcomed the harmonization: "If there are going to be two referees, they will have to agree on the rules."

When a team of international auditors went to the Montreal, Saint John, and Winnipeg centres in late October and early November 1994, they found a chaotic system. Centre staff were unclear if they should be listening to the Bureau of Biologics, the national Red Cross, or the FDA, they reported. "There was evidence of inconsistencies which led to confusion." The auditors were critical of the inspection team sent from the Red Cross headquarters. "However well intentioned and committed the National team are, it was clear from our audits that as a unit they were, at best, ineffective." Directives had been sent from headquarters that "made unreasonable demands for rapid, excessive, and at times, ill-conceived change." If these changes were to be made, they would lead to breaches in so-called good manufacturing practices. The autocratic approach from the national Red Cross led to frustration, bemusement, and resentment. "It must be assumed that the national office are oblivious to the problems they are causing."

The auditors, working on behalf of the Krever inquiry, found many major shortcomings at the centres they inspected. They listed fourteen at the Montreal centre, twenty at Saint John, and twenty-four at Winnipeg. Nearly all had been missed by previous Canadian inspections.

Both Red Cross and federal officials had repeatedly argued that there was no danger to the public and the deficiencies were not a threat to the integrity of the Canadian system. But if nothing else, an already battered blood system had taken another public mauling and critics were pointing to the debacle as another reason control should be taken from the Red Cross.

Maung Aye, the Red Cross national director of blood services, said in an interview earlier in 1994 that he hoped the centres would soon be up to FDA scratch. He characterized the FDA rules as a hangover from the 1970s when the Americans were importing questionable plasma from all over the world.

That may be, but the FDA inspections cannot be dismissed by Canadian authorities. There is brave talk about harmonization. But don't the Americans hold all the cards, since it is Canadian blood flowing south that requires processing? Kent Foster, assistant deputy minister of the Health Protection Branch, disagreed with that view in September 1994. "My discussions with the FDA on the question of harmonization have been on the basis of 'We like a couple of things you're doing as well.' That's harmonization. They are not demanding that we harmonize in any particular way. But to ship source plasma to them for fractionation, the Red Cross must meet their regulations."

The danger remains that the Americans could change their mind, get tough, and block all Canadian plasma from entering the United States for processing. That's a concern of the Canadian Hemophilia Society, which says that for twelve years the Red Cross and Ottawa have known of the need for FDA-licensing. There are no guarantees for the current exemption from U.S. licensing rules. What now allows most Canadian plasma across the border licence-free is the grandfathered long-term processing contract between the Red Cross and Cutter. What if that agreement is terminated and the Red Cross still does not meet FDA standards? Would Canadian plasma be stopped from crossing the border? It's a sticky little problem we can only hope does not arise until Canadian authorities get their act together.

Perhaps some soothsayer should have warned the Caesar of the Canadian blood system to beware the Ides of March. Not only was March 15, 1994, the controversial deadline for acceptance by tainted blood victims of the provincial assistance package, the Red Cross was startled by another bombshell at the Krever inquiry in March. The second month of hearings was just under way when David Harvey, a lawyer representing blood-transfused victims, revealed the Toronto regional centre had stored 175,000 frozen samples of blood taken from donations made between November 1984 and October 1985.

That was a critical time in the evolution of the bad blood scandal, and the samples, if properly catalogued, might be a storehouse of vital information. In November 1984, the decision was made to switch to heat-treated blood products. By October 1985, heat-treated products had been introduced and donor screening through the ELISA test had just begun in at least some provinces. If the samples were tested for HIV, it could tell much about the status of Red Cross blood donors at the time. More important, it could provide a way to track down HIV-infected donors and recipients, some of whom still might not know they carried the deadly virus.

Harvey raised the matter as he was questioning Dr. Philip Berger of Toronto. Berger had earlier opined that if a breach of confidentiality would save a life, then it was a justifiable breach. The lawyer pointed out that the Red Cross had not gone back to see if the samples were HIV-positive and traced them through the system.

"If that's true, they should start testing this morning and identify those samples that are infected and ensure the recipients are aware of it," said Berger. "I'm kind of shocked, with all the publicity and everything else that's gone on, that there are samples that could result in identifying someone who was unaware they were transfused."

The Red Cross explanation is that the samples had been collected by a doctor working at the centre who was interested in studying post-transfusion hepatitis. Samples were saved from all donors at the Toronto centre for six months. The donors were told, the Red Cross maintains, that the samples were being retained for hepatitis B tests.

Maung Aye says the "hullabaloo" posed an "ethical dilemma," and the issue was turned over by the Red Cross to an ethics committee for an opinion.

"We could test them so we can tell the recipients, but the biggest problem is that this blood was taken at a time before we had announced we were going to do HIV testing. So these were taken from people who didn't know they would be tested for HIV. You know how sensitive the situation is in the public. You just can't go out and test anybody's blood for HIV just because you feel like it," said Aye.

"Although it's okay to do the testing for the recipient, what do you do about the donor? My hands are doubly tied because by public health law, if you get a positive result, I have to notify the public health authorities; and if you notify the authorities, you have to notify the donor before the authorities. Some people who are infected don't want to know, and some people who are infected have other recourse over this ten-year period, to determine where and when they want to get tested. They didn't come to the Red Cross to get tested for HIV."

Was this an artificial dilemma? In October 1985, the Red Cross changed its policy to explicitly tell donors all blood was tested "as a matter of course" for hepatitis B, syphilis, and the AIDS-related virus. But after May 1984 there had been an "implied consent" that donations might be tested. "Donors must be informed that tests are being done but specific consents are not required to perform testing," the Red Cross said then. So, testing for HIV would be permitted either generally or specifically.

The Red Cross response wasn't fast enough for the blood-transfused people Harvey represented, or for the Canadian Hemophilia Society. Both groups wrote Prime Minister Jean Chrétien calling for testing. The CHS claimed gross negligence was involved and the Red Cross licence should be suspended. When federal authorities declined to act, saying they had no jurisdiction, the HIV-T group requested help from the

City of Toronto medical officer. "Lives have been lost already to inaction and delays while governments pondered procedural and juris-dictional niceties," complained Jerry Freise. Once again, when faced with a challenge, the blood system seemed temporarily handcuffed.

The ethics committee, chaired by Dr. Margaret Somerville of McGill University's Centre for Medicine, Ethics, and Law, reported in August 1994, estimating that between eighteen to fifty-nine undis-covered cases of HIV-infection might be found by testing the samples. There was an ethical requirement to test so that transfusion recipients, and their "at risk" partners, could be warned they were exposed to HIV.

For infected donors, it was another story. Notification was not eth-ically required, would constitute compulsory testing, and was not justified, the committee concluded. But a light switched on in the minds of the ethicists. Perhaps some of the donors would actually want to know if they were HIV-positive. After all, they have "at risk" partners, too. The committee recommended the Red Cross provide a service, such as a toll-free phone line, that would let donors choose to find out their status.

An old dilemma had resurfaced. Ontario law required the names of all persons who were confirmed HIV-positive to be reported to public health authorities. But the ethical experts recommended that the Red Cross not report to the government the names of HIV-positive donors found through the testing.

The impasse echoed a debate that had occurred in 1985. On October 10 that year, Dr. A. S. Macpherson, medical officer of health for Toronto, noted that a similar procedure could be used for HIV-positive donors as was already employed with syphilitic donors. In that situation, the Red Cross obtained the names of the donors' personal physicians so they could follow up and counsel their patients. If there were delays in pursuing this course, Macpherson suggested, public health should become involved. He chastised the Red Cross for resist-ing legal notification. The Red Cross "is creating a dangerous double standard by providing a route for HTLV-III identification through blood donation which offers an opportunity to avoid appropriate follow-up." Macpherson said he realized a positive test could create "uncertainties and dilemmas," but criticized unnecessary delays in the planning and implementation of donor notification.

At the heart of this continuing debate is the question of whether individual privacy or the health and safety of the public is to be paramount. Some HIV-infected individuals have faced charges under the Criminal Code for having unprotected sex with unwitting partners. If governments or the Red Cross knew a donor was infectious and failed to warn that person, would they bear the moral or legal responsibility if a partner became infected?

The Canadian AIDS Society went to court in 1994 to stop the names from being handed over to Ontario health authorities, arguing that step would infringe on privacy and constitute compulsory testing. Ontario Judge Doug Carruthers ruled that the names should be turned over. The issue was not the rights of a few individuals but "the health and well-being of society," he wrote. The Canadian AIDS Society vowed to appeal.

BOB PEDERSEN

Bob Pedersen, father of two hemophiliac sons, served as president of the Canadian Hemophilia Society during the troubling years 1986 and 1987. He argues that members of the medical community must make themselves more open to the public.

"They can't live in the world of the God complex any longer," says Pedersen, whose stature and blond hair affirm his Scandinavian roots. "They have to come down to earth and say: 'This isn't a great mystery, folks. We're just body plumbers. Some of us are highly skilled body plumbers, but we're all body plumbers. Some of us don't like the smell, so we're mind plumbers.' And if you have to use fancier communication than that, it's not to make it accessible, but inaccessible. And there's only two reasons for doing that: to cut your losses because you keep people in ignorance, or because you're really not doing that great a job and you want to keep people in ignorance. But in either event, you want to keep people in ignorance."

Bob Pederson says a lesson of the past is that the medical system needs to be scrutinized by non-medical people. The worst thing to have, he argues, is a profession that monitors itself. "If any profession is shrouded in such mystique that an average intelligent person can't understand it, then that profession should be banned. Because if you can't put your technical terms in common language for all to understand, they're not valid terms. They're voodoo. They're magic.

"If you hold yourself above the common man, all you're saying is that you don't hold the common man's life to be of any value."

Pedersen says he's frightened by the current preoccupation with cost-cutting in the health system. "Every Canadian is exposed in that situation. That means your medical group, your ministry of health, says: 'First look at the dollars, look at how many people are likely to die, and then toss a coin.' That's the quality of their decision-making. And that's scary.

"Government has a tendency to reflect the prejudices of the community. We saw that when the gay community came down with AIDS. 'It's a gay disease. Let them die. They're abnormal or inferior. Somehow they are less than people. So we can keep our voters happy by letting the gays die.' So then, hemophiliacs come along. 'These are defective people anyway, and Canadians shouldn't be too concerned the blood system murdered them.'

"But where does it stop? We're getting to the point that just about any Canadian's life is dismissible by the government. And we're not sure under what terms it is dismissible. It seems to be getting pretty flimsy when if you have sex with your wife you're at risk, and sorry about your luck. Or if your children catch it through the umbilical cord, don't have kids. Sorry, but bad luck.

"That's a kind of arrogance, which I'm sure is not intentional. What is prompting this decision-making? Money is coming before philosophy and the value of human life. If somebody, the hemophilia community or somebody else, doesn't argue strongly for this situation to be altered, there is nobody else."

Pedersen elegantly frames his undeniable anger in a reasoned way. In fact, he prides himself on his negotiating skills, an ability to bring people together in consensus. But there's a lingering sadness in having seen many friends and co-workers die from AIDS.

"I think there are a lot of heroes who are never going to be recognized in the Hemophilia Society. There is a real sadness that some of these people are even feeling a lack of respect these days. I saw people who were sick, who were really in rough shape, fighting to do things on behalf of other hemophiliacs. Everything from players at the national level to the guy who said, 'Yes, I'll come and help you with your charity bingo,' and died two weeks later. We don't know our heroes; we don't recognize our heroes; and we do a very poor job of celebrating what we have accomplished. And the Canadian Hemophilia Society has accomplished things that no other group has accomplished anywhere in the world. I think that sometime, somewhere, that needs celebrating."

Chapter 16

WHO'S IN CHARGE?

"We'll live through it, and we'll use it.
We won't let our children die in vain."

DENISE ORIEUX, MAY 1994

The people who ran the Canadian blood system in the 1980s can move along to other ventures and put their part in the tainted blood affair behind them. Many have. But for those who suffer from the system's breakdown, there is no end to the tragedy.

Gloria Ann Smith, whose son Scott died on July 6, 1992, reminded the Krever inquiry of that lingering pain in March 1994 in an emotional conclusion to the testimony of three mothers with infected children.

"It didn't end in 1992," she said. "It still goes on. We're reminded of it every day. We still haven't been able to mourn properly. There's always something coming out about it. I just hope this commission can get to the bottom of it, so it will never happen again."

The system in the 1980s was slow to react and confused. It featured a timid consumer group, an arrogant monopoly, an indecisive profession that "buries its mistakes," a regulator lacking the tools or the will to do its job, and a group of cost-conscious governments paying the bills. Taken together, it was a rickety structure. And this shaky construction led to disaster.

Is this too harsh an indictment of the blood system as it existed in the mid-1980s? Either as donors or as recipients, we must remember that we are all likely to play a role in the blood system at some point. As consumers of health services, we need to know how the key players of the blood system failed.

Despite a lead time of a year to two years in the spread of the AIDS epidemic, Canada did not escape the pattern already set in the United States. Any head start, any lesson we could have learned from the American experience, was squandered. The introduction of heat-treated products, the questioning of blood donors, and testing for the virus were all debated here just as they had been in the United States — and in each case Canada introduced these measures later.

The public face of the blood authorities was reassurance, that everything was under control, but behind the scenes there lurked indifference and chaos. Had the public known just how confused the authorities were, perhaps they wouldn't have been as complacent. Some officials spoke of the potential for public panic, suggesting that the judgment of Canadians was not to be trusted. This is the arrogance of the oligarchy. Today, the excuse is made that no one knew how to protect the public. Yet we know that some doctors, even before HIV was identified, saw the danger and did advise measures that shielded people in their care. Some experts who have looked at the system in the 1990s say it really hasn't changed all that much.

The public halo the Red Cross has worn makes that institution all the more difficult to tackle when it has blundered. Tainted blood has been the toughest test of this angelic aura, forcing the organization to put a good deal of its resources into a costly public relations campaign to repair the damage.

Some who dealt with the Red Cross in the 1980s have a less than rosy view of the organization. Former employees who were once mainstays of the blood program openly describe it as dysfunctional, a frustrating place to work. One criticism is that the Red Cross has too much on its plate — international relief programs, water safety, social activities, and the blood program — and that board members with little or no knowledge of how the blood system works end up making vital decisions about a "dangerous drug."

Dr. Gail Rock, a former medical director, biochemist, and internationally renowned researcher, sarcastically calls her onetime employer "The Great Red Mother." Rock was fired by the Red Cross in 1988 and won a partial victory in a wrongful dismissal suit six years later. Her suit had been met by a trumped-up countersuit for "breach of duty." By the time Rock left, her research — which she says might have made Canada self-sufficient in clotting factors at a critical time — had come to a halt. She had worked on production of synthetic or recombinant Factor VIII in the early 1980s. By 1994, recombinant clotting factor was standard treatment in Canada. The country might not only have been self-sufficient but even an exporter had her work succeeded. But she was told to forget artificially produced Factor VIII, told it was an impossible dream. Rock also developed a process that would increase threefold the yields of Factor VIII from plasma. The Red Cross held a patent on the process but never used it and would not advance funds for further work. She says it might have been a financial windfall for the Red Cross.

There were many departures of experienced professionals from the Red Cross, voluntary or otherwise, in the late 1980s. Bureaucracy was rampant, there were few medical experts at senior levels, and there was little local autonomy. Employees were frustrated by autocratic management and the sluggishness of the national office in responding to emergencies. The foot-dragging by the national Red Cross in screening high-risk donors was a case in point.

As HIV was spreading through the blood system, the seventeen regional directors seemed to recognize the threat well ahead of national officers. Many pressed for more specific questioning of donors and some advised use of less risky alternative blood products. These warnings were ignored. The national office said constantly "to all of us in the field that there is no proven evidence that AIDS is transmitted by blood transfusions," says one former medical director. "The

Red Cross is not a democracy" was another pet theme. It was an odd line for an outfit that was supposed to be community-based.

Outsiders found it frustrating to deal with an organization that would not listen to their concerns and ideas. Bill Mindell, chair of the factor products committee of Hemophilia Ontario, had hard words for the blood transfusion service in December 1985, after heat-treated product was distributed and testing of donors had begun. He spoke of the "chaos, arrogance, and incompetence" of the Red Cross.

"A great deal of damage was done to (especially young) hemophiliacs and the general Canadian population by unnecessary exposure to the AIDS virus," he wrote. "I think it is now recognized by many professionals close to the AIDS issue in Canada that the leadership (and I use the term loosely) of the Canadian Red Cross Blood Transfusion Service simply did not rise to the challenge. As well, the decision-making apparatus of the government or the Canadian Blood Committee didn't or couldn't act when necessary, and left the responsibility for action in this emergency in the hands of the people least capable of doing anything about it."

Mindell said then he would prefer some public health agency to have overriding authority to take action. The Red Cross has amply demonstrated that they would not protect public health. "They are much more concerned with their production schedules for a product — a sort of factory mentality." His call for a public agency echoes the conclusion reached by some who had worked inside the Red Cross, and still rings true.

Time has made Mindell more philosophical. "It's not good enough to scapegoat a couple of Red Cross individuals. It was the system at fault. The system failed."

The monopoly structure of the system may have had some benefits to Canadians. Unlike the United States, this country does not have numbers of profit-oriented players with varying attitudes to the purchasing of blood from paid donors.

But monopoly has had its drawbacks, too, especially when it comes to sharing information and power. The Red Cross has held back relevant contract information from the taxpayer-funded Canadian Blood Agency. The feeble Bureau of Biologics has been virtually ignored and has continually deferred to Red Cross expertise. The result is that decisions about the source and price of blood products have been made in secret and without public accountability. These industrial secrets could prevent Canadians from getting the best products at the best possible cost.

With a virtual monopoly on the information, the Red Cross wields a heavy stick over other agencies, including the CBA. It negotiates and signs the contracts and thereby has substantial influence over what products are to be used. Although Red Cross officials have maintained in the past that choice of product is the role of the treating physician, doctors and clinicians have received their contract and cost information from the Red Cross. When it comes to blood products, the Red Cross is effectively policeman, prosecutor, and judge. Or, more precisely — collector, middleman, distributor, and, to a degree, prescriber. It then hoofs the bills over to the Canadian public.

Another kind of control in the system is less obvious. There is a limit to the scientific expertise available in the complex field of blood and blood products, so the players often shift roles. Thus, Wark Boucher, who was with the Bureau of Biologics during the critical period of the mid-1980s, now works for the Red Cross. Michael O'Shaughnessy, who did the first HIV tests on Canadian hemophiliacs while with the federal Laboratory Centre for Disease Control, heads a Vancouver AIDS project that relies on federal funds. Gail Rock, fired from the Red Cross, now works for the Bureau of Human Prescription Drugs, a part of the federal Health Protection Branch. The Canadian Blood Agency has looked to the Red Cross as a source of staff. The dependence of individuals on their current employer or funder might help to insulate or protect these institutions if they are called before the public inquiry.

There was little doubt in the 1980s as to who was the Red Cross blood boss. Roger Perrault was national director of the Blood

Transfusion Service during this period. Perrault, who was on Canadian Hemophilia Society letterhead as an honorary life member until his suspension in May 1994, has been described by former employees of the Red Cross as an intimidating man. "If you stood up for your rights, he dealt with you better," said one colleague. "But he felt challenged by bright and articulate people." Some see Perrault in a more sympathetic light. He changed over time after losing battles to politicians and Red Cross board members who were jealous of the attention given the blood transfusion service, they say. "Roger tried hard at the beginning, but he was battering against a brick wall." Eventually, Perrault stopped fighting and moved on. He is now president of the Industrial Biotechnology Association of Canada.

Some reasons why the Red Cross failed to act more quickly in the mid-1980s may never be known. Two of Perrault's most senior deputies, John Derrick and Derek Naylor, took the logic for their decisions to the grave. Both died in the late 1980s.

Perrault, too, reported to his boss, George Weber, the Red Cross secretary-general and chief executive during the crisis period. Weber, who has now gone on to the International Red Cross, apparently had a surprising lack of interest in the blood program.

Richard Huntsman, medical director of the Newfoundland Red Cross centre, told the Krever hearings that he was surprised that Weber would often visit the St. John's Red Cross building but never its blood centre. Huntsman told of an occasion when he asked Weber about sabbaticals for medical directors to upgrade their skills. "His reply, I remember distinctly, was 'When I give it to my water safety instructors, I will give it to the medical directors.' I did not think that showed ability to manage professional staff."

Huntsman also noted that Perrault could be intimated by Weber. When a nurse retired at the St. John's centre after twenty-five years' service, Perrault sent a glowing telegram to Huntsman. Later, Perrault called Huntsman and told him not to read the message. "I said, why not? It was a wonderful telegram. He said, 'I'm not asking your opinion,' and we got the Perrault authoritarian treatment, which I respect." Perrault explained the telegram had to be withdrawn because Weber's name was not included on it. "I was aware then that there were influences at work above him," Huntsman said.

Perrault's reaction to allegations that the Red Cross failed to act for public safety in the mid-1980s has been a hand-washing of responsibility. "We followed exactly what the public health authorities told us to do to the letter," he told the *Canadian Medical Association Journal* in 1990. Yet the December 1984 inventory of blood products suggests it was the Red Cross that chose the May 1, 1985, implementation date for distribution of heat-treated concentrates, even before input from the other involved parties.

David Page, past president of the Canadian Hemophilia Society, says the 1984 consensus conference shows the Red Cross got everyone to agree to its own timetable. "Once people knew what was going on, everybody was involved, even the Hemophilia Society. It was an excellent way not to make a decision, not to admit that everything that had been said up until then was most likely wrong. We could now get everybody together and invite them into a new plan that would bring in the new products but would do it on a timetable that would make everybody as guilty as everybody else."

Public health officials certainly seem to have relied heavily for advice upon the Red Cross blood supply experts. Dr. Alexander S. Macpherson, medical officer of health for the City of Toronto between 1981 and 1988, testifying at the Krever inquiry, recalled a set of sample responses prepared as answers to questions from the media.

One anticipated question asked about the safety of the blood system. The response was firm and unqualified: there is no evidence of the blood supply causing AIDS — no reports of AIDS cases due to transfusion. This was a proposed response in August 1983, well after proven cases of contamination through blood products and transfusions had shown up in the United States and in Canada.

Should elective surgery be cancelled, another question asked. "Definitely not" was the response, months after medical advisors to the Canadian Hemophilia Society had called for deferral of elective surgery. "There is no evidence that blood is any less safe than prior to the appearance of AIDS."

"Quite clearly," Macpherson told the inquiry, "these answers came from the Red Cross." The Great Red Mother syndrome was alive and flourishing. There was no reason to disbelieve the answers, Macpherson felt. There was a known risk in the United States, but no way of knowing if the risk was greater or less or the same in Canada. "Our view was the prevailing Canadian view, which was the risk was low."

The bad blood catastrophe may have harmed the reputation of the Red Cross but has not diminished its arrogance. While Douglas Lindores, the Red Cross secretary-general, goes on public-speaking tours to defend his agency, the victims and their families wait in vain for the apology that would salve their wounds. Lindores blames the media for sensationalizing what is a sensational story. It will induce patients to start refusing blood transfusions, he says. But independent experts are cautioning against over-use of blood products. With periodic fits of petulance, the Red Cross threatens to quit the blood system unless things are done its way. Its leaders would prefer not to be held accountable to the public for their decisions. Critics, including former employees, say that as the Red Cross has adopted a more corporate identity, it is losing its humanitarian focus.

In a speech to the Canadian Club in Toronto in November 1994, Lindores said the Red Cross decision to proceed with a blood fractionation plant over the protests of consumers and the provincial governments showed leadership. "The decision reflects one important lesson the Canadian Red Cross Society has learned from the tragedy of the eighties — the determination to exercise our leadership in everything we can, alone if necessary, to provide a safe and secure supply of blood and blood products to the Canadian health system," he said.

If this determination to assert its dominance is all the Red Cross learned from the 1980s, then heaven help us!

* * *

One would like to believe that when the crisis came in the early to mid-1980s, doctors who were expert in hemophilia took special pains to defend and inform their client population. Unfortunately, this did not happen. A sense of urgency was lacking. Most hemophiliacs were going ahead with their lives, not paying attention to less-than-explicit advice coming from various quarters. The treating physicians seemed either confused, complacent, or uninformed. The general message was not to change — that HIV infection was not a widespread problem.

"Nobody was fighting for better blood," says Bob O'Neill of the CHS. He blames a series of missteps that occurred over two to three years. "You can't say there was one critical meeting where everything was screwed up. It was a series of indecisions leading up to a climax of indecision."

O'Neill believes in retrospect the hematologists realized they had made mistakes. At a meeting in February 1988, they stood up against the Canadian Blood Committee — the agency of the provinces — and insisted upon the purchase of the more expensive but safer new products. "The hematologists for the first time took the side of the hemophilia community."

One has to wonder why the pilot of the system, the federal Bureau of Biologics, was not more active at the time Canadian blood was being contaminated. The Bureau seems to have roused itself drowsily from sleep only once in a while, dozing off again for long stretches. From August 1982, when it warned the Red Cross to watch out for infected hemophiliacs, until November 16, 1984, when it ordered that heat-treated blood products be obtained, the Bureau made virtually no intervention. Caution in the use of blood products was not advised despite evidence that the immune systems of many hemophiliacs were under stress. There was no apparent move to check whether heat-treated products, already licensed for Canadian use, and prepared for use against other viral contaminants, could also be employed to offset the danger of this new virus.

Why, for example, did the government respond so slowly to

Michael O'Shaughnessy's dramatic findings in the summer of 1984 concerning the HIV infection rate among hemophiliacs? The Laboratory Centre for Disease Control reported to the assistant deputy minister of the Health Protection Branch, as did the Bureau of Biologics, the federal regulator of blood products. Yet no one in that branch seems to have taken these startling results and treated them with the urgency they demanded.

After its recommendation of heat-treated products only, the Bureau disappeared again for some time, defending the dry-heated, distributed products until caught short again by the late infections in Western Canada of seven more hemophiliacs. Where were they when the system needed close supervision and a watchful eye?

To David Page, the federal government abdicated its responsibility to the Red Cross. "The Bureau of Biologics never really regulated and still is not sufficiently regulating the blood system," he says. "They didn't have the expertise or the knowledge or the personnel to do it. What they really did was let the Red Cross regulate itself. When there was an issue that came forward, they would rely on the advice of the Red Cross. So long as the Red Cross was saying there was no proof that there was HIV in the blood system, the Bureau didn't have the resources, or the will, to question them."

Page says the Red Cross was not ultimately responsible for protecting the blood supply. But it had filled this role since the 1940s and the Bureau had stepped away from its obligation. "Certainly, no pharmaceutical company would have been able to get away with the same kind of freedom. You just wouldn't find a Sandoz or a CIBA-Geigy regulating itself when it came to drugs. Obviously, the federal government has to play its role correctly, which it's not doing."

An international safety audit conducted for the Krever inquiry in the fall of 1994 shows little has changed. "The Bureau of Biologics is under-resourced and has not taken a leadership role in assuring safety of the blood supply," it concluded. Canada has not been optimally served by the regulators. "The evidence in support of this conclusion is overwhelming and it is difficult not to conclude that, as a consequence, significant and inappropriate quality deficiencies may exist in some parts of the Canadian Red Cross." Regular, comprehensive inspections with timely follow-up are needed, the auditors said. Astoundingly, when the auditors went to make what is perhaps the most important review in the Bureau's history, they had limited access to many of the most senior staff. These people were away on other business, on holidays, or recently retired.

Regulatory failure is not unique to Canada. Page was told by a European transfusion service director that the unearthing of the UB Plasma scandal was just a stroke of luck and didn't happen because regulators were doing their job. "Screening and viral inactivation are excellent today. The problem is you may have human error, or companies that want to cut corners and save a bit of money, companies that are dishonest and criminal as was UB Plasma, and nobody really checking. That's where the danger is. We've been saying that to the federal government for the last year and a half. That's one part of the checks and balances that needs to be strengthened."

Profit-driven, the manufacturers stood to lose a lot of money from a switch-over to heat-treated products. Non-heat-processed stocks would have to be destroyed, and already consumer mistrust and the return to alternatives like cryoprecipitate had proven costly. In the United States, some hemophiliacs have undertaken a class action suit against four American-based manufacturers — Alpha, Armour, Baxter-Hyland, and Miles-Cutter — saying the companies aggressively marketed their products while downplaying the significant risk of viral contamination. The group has also included the National Hemophilia Foundation in its suit, alleging it conspired with the manufacturers to promote use of the products while it was funded by the fractionators. In Canada, those kinds of actions have been largely averted by the federal and provincial compensation packages.

Of course, manufacturers also had an incentive not to lose all their customers. Dead clients don't use your product.

Why did companies like Cutter and Armour promise the Red

Cross so much more than they could deliver in 1985? Did they want to nail down the Canadian contract even though they knew they would not be able to meet the demand? If so, that is a kind of corporate dishonesty that cannot be tolerated.

The blood system today, in part because of the 1980s disaster, is a backdrop for feuding principalities led by battling MBAs. Douglas Lindores of the Red Cross, William Dobson of the Canadian Blood Agency, and Dann Michols, executive director of the Health Department's drugs directorate, are all MBAs who have emerged from bureaucratic backgrounds.

The Krever inquiry's safety audit released in November 1994 concluded that while the Canadian blood supply is no less safe than that of other developed countries, the system needs to be restructured to eliminate conflicts and to define responsibilities. The report particularly noted the "openly antagonistic" relations between the Red Cross and the Canadian Blood Agency.

If this and other deficiencies are not corrected, the report warned, there is "significant potential risk to the safety of the Canadian blood supply in future years."

Lindores and Dobson agree on at least one thing—the lack of clarity in the Canadian blood system has caused confusion and conflict. Maung Aye, national director of blood services for the Red Cross, aptly describes it as a body with two heads. Just about everything else has been in dispute. It's an unseemly quarrel that features two of the main players in the blood system squaring off in a very public battle.

They have even fought over who actually owns the blood that is given freely by Canadian volunteers. The Red Cross has set its lawyers to work and they have come up with an opinion that it owns the blood collected through the monopoly collection centres and has the right to decide how it is used. Lindores has said donated blood is "held in trust" for Canadians while it is in the possession of the Red Cross. The Red Cross says polls show a majority of donors agree with that position. Aye says the whole debate makes him sick. "Who owns a donated heart or a liver?" he asks rhetorically.

A request to the Red Cross for a policy statement on ownership of blood brought a bizarre response — a newspaper clipping and a seven-line paragraph. The statement says there was no connection between ownership and the infection of blood products in the early 1980s. The two issues are "not in any way related." But, surely, if you "own" a hazardous product which you collect and distribute, and which subsequently causes injury and death, there must be a relationship. You must have obligations to ensure that the product you own and distribute to others is safe. The Red Cross appears to claim rights on one hand but expects to duck responsibility on the other.

The Canadian Hemophilia Society argues that volunteer-donated plasma should be publicly owned, not become the property of an organization with no public accountability. Page says the Red Cross runs a "decent" blood collection system, although donor recruitment could be better. But the blood system must be more than just a milk cow for the Red Cross. It must be accountable to the public.

Meanwhile, the Canadian Blood Agency, the sparsely staffed bureaucracy that pays the bills, has had problems asserting itself. The CBA has been compelled to rely on Red Cross information and has even been prevented from seeing the Red Cross–manufacturer deals. Contract partners thus plead confidentiality and expect the agency to cough up the dough.

The pitched public battle over a $150-million Canadian blood fractionation plant has been the most gaping wound in the CBA–Red Cross relationship. The Red Cross defied a CBA directive not to proceed in a partnership with Miles-Cutter, and in June 1994 was given a green light by a blue-ribbon panel appointed by the provinces. The proposed Halifax-area plant would produce albumin, immunoglobulin, and intermediate-purity Factor VIII. Anything surplus to Canadian needs (most Canadian hemophiliacs now use ultra-high-purity products) would be turned over to

Miles to supply foreign clients. The plant would be run by a new fractionation company at arm's-length from the Red Cross and would create four hundred jobs.

Aye says the plant capacity would be over 800,000 litres of plasma a year, twice the available Canadian supply, so half the plasma to be processed would be imported. After each run, the plant would be "bombed"— sterilized so that Canadian products would not be contaminated by any imported stuff. "What that does for us is increase the economies of scale, because the more you produce, the cost per unit goes down," says Aye. "We can put our cryoprecipitate through and it offsets the cost of the other products. This will be a showcase, so quality-wise we have to be as good as the best plants."

The Red Cross argues that processing Canadian-source plasma in Canada will mean self-sufficiency in blood products. But Dobson has maintained that if the United States is the most efficient place to fractionate Canadian blood, this will not undermine national self-sufficiency. It's an interesting reversal from the bad old days of Connaught.

While the provinces had been critical for political and economic reasons — some wanted the plant in their own backyard — the Canadian Hemophilia Society view is that the project should have been held off until Judge Krever filed his inquiry report. It is conceivable, after all, that the Red Cross could be elbowed out of the blood business altogether.

Many hemophiliacs resent the idea that the Red Cross, which they hold responsible for the catastrophe of the 1980s, is being publicly rewarded by being permitted to establish the plant that will be the centrepiece of its empire. It is a bitter kick in the teeth.

Dobson told the Krever inquiry in early 1994 that there is no consensus between the Red Cross and the Canadian Blood Agency on the roles each should play. "The problem arises if that role [of the CBA] is not accepted by the major player in the blood system." In turn, Lindores told the inquiry the Red Cross would do its best to cooperate with the CBA but "will not consider itself bound by its directives."

The Red Cross was outraged when the Agency trimmed, without negotiation, 2 per cent from its budget seven months into one fiscal year. Lindores tried to shift blame for the failed FDA inspections to the Agency by noting a delay in payment of $7 million needed to implement FDA-required "good manufacturing practices." Dobson has held back $1.7 million in funding for the Red Cross's long-awaited computer because the estimated cost, initially set at $10.3 million, had swollen within six months by another $5 million. The huge increase suggested trouble was brewing, Dobson said.

The Red Cross also spurned a CBA proposal to start a joint insurance fund. The idea was that both the Agency and the Red Cross would put money into a fund that could be used to pay claims when people are injured by the blood system. "We were never able to sell this idea to the Red Cross, because the whole relationship problem, our mandate, our legitimacy, our right to exist and do what we are supposed to do, as set out by the ministers, that was felt to take precedence," complained Dobson.

The CBA and the Red Cross even have differing views on such a basic concept as safety. Lindores, for example, agreed before the Krever inquiry with the notion that "safety is paramount." Dobson's response was more qualified. "While safety is paramount," he said, "the question is how much safety can government afford and at what point and who is prepared to draw the line on where the money sort of runs out." It's the most difficult question in health care today, he added.

That's the kind of remark that sets off alarm bells in health advocates. If the public faces a peril like AIDS, how much trust should be invested in a bureaucracy that says safety is okay, just as long as it doesn't cost too much.

Dr. Philip Berger, also testifying before Krever, summed up the issue of taxpayer cost versus public benefit. "People should understand that governments and people in positions of power in governments make decisions regularly, with respect to allocation of funds, that can result in illness, injury, and death." He pointed out that for two years it had been recommended that every resident of Canada receive hepatitis B vaccination.

"The Ontario government has no universal hepatitis B immunization program, even though it is a preventative measure that will prevent injury and death. That's a decision the government made of not allocating funds to that program. How do we as a society decide where to put money? Is it worth $10 million to pick up one HIV-infected person who might be unaware of it, even unaware of having had a blood transfusion ten years ago? I don't know the answer, but I think it's important that the public knows that these decisions are being made and there is no public debate about it."

There is a message for the volunteer health sector today in what happened to the Canadian Hemophilia Society at the time of crisis in the mid-1980s. Stand apart and look objectively at the facts. Investigate even the "one-in-a-million" ideas that are being rejected by your professionals. Don't be afraid to question. Don't allow yourselves to become docile and dependent. Trust no one. Follow your own instincts and use common sense.

Today the CHS is paying the price of reticence and complacency in the early eighties. Back then, a few members were clearly unhappy about the glacial pace of the Society in defending the interests of hemophiliacs. But they were a vocal minority. That docility has led to rage and dissension in the ranks that continues to this day. Some hemophiliacs, angry because they believe the Society failed them, washed their hands of it completely. There are accusations that members have been taken in by whitewash and revisionist history. There is frustration that executives have lost touch with the grassroots. No consumer organization can afford that kind of internal strife. The situation is even worse in the United States, where some members of the Committee of Ten Thousand (representing the number of American hemophiliacs infected) have split from the National Hemophilia Foundation and are taking legal action against it.

In the eighties, dependency upon the Red Cross and the doctors had eroded the Society's role of consumer advocate. Hemophiliacs and their well-meaning kin were left starry-eyed by rubbing shoulders with the country's medical and bureaucratic elite. There was a large body of opinion — which still exists to a degree — that criticism would backfire. Either the Red Cross would punish hemophiliacs for raising embarrassing questions about the quality and safety of blood, or donors might stop giving the commodity that was so precious.

What we have today is a blood system that still lacks effective coordination and features deep-rooted hostility and suspicions among the key players — the Red Cross, the Canadian Blood Agency, the Bureau of Biologics, and the consumers. There is still, for instance, no clearly defined emergency response system. The UB Plasma affair showed that despite the lessons of the last decade, responsibility for safety and coordination of efforts are ill-defined for the various players in the system.

The half-billion-dollar question is, Was anyone really taking charge of the situation, and is anyone today? The answer, then and now, is no. There were flaws in the whole blood regulation and distribution framework. Bob O'Neill, a CHS employee at that critical time, says the whole system was muddied by a lack of clear direction. "Nobody was at the helm."

The theme was emphasized when the Canadian Hemophilia Society made its case for compensation for victims from the governments, Red Cross, and other participants in the system. "During the critical years of HIV transmission, there seemed to be no mechanism to promptly address problems of safety and supply," the compensation committee said in its 1988 brief to the federal government. "It seemed that no one agency wanted to take ultimate responsibility for guarding the safety of the system. In other words, if the blood-product technology was a *Titanic* and HIV was the iceberg, who, then was serving as the lookout?"

* * *

The need for a specialized governing agency to oversee the system and set policy has become a centrepiece of reform for many groups. The Hemophilia Society has said it would prefer to see a non-profit, government-funded agency replace the Red Cross as the lead organization, to assume control over the amount and type of products to be purchased, and do quality and efficacy testing as well.

A single, authoritative governing agency with the necessary resources to make informed decisions was recommended in late 1994 by the Canadian Public Health Association, an independent voluntary association. What stands out in the CPHA brief is the proposition that the public and consumers be given equal standing in that body with the suppliers, prescribers, and funders of the system. As a first principle, the association calls for consumer orientation. "The ultimate 'consumer' is the recipient of blood and blood products — the assumer of risk," its says. "All aspects of the national blood system should revolve around, and serve, consumer needs." This attention to the consumer has so far been rejected by the hierarchies of the powers that be.

Some are of the opinion that the Canadian Blood Agency should be given control. But the reputation of government bureaucracies makes some people nervous about this option.

Mr. Justice Horace Krever's interim report on Canada's troubled blood system was made public on February 24, 1995. There was little immediate solace in it for people affected by bad blood in the last decade. They will have to wait for the final report to see if their grievances will be redressed. Given the rapacious nature of AIDS, many will not live to see the inquiry results.

Still, Krever confronted several failings of the system in his forty-three interim recommendations. He called for a restructuring to eliminate conflict and define responsibilities for safety. He warned that the blood system is still at risk from unknown contaminants, and called upon the Bureau of Biologics and the Red Cross to clean up their acts in inspection and correction of operating deficiencies. Dedicated, competent inspectors who understand both the blood industry and good manufacturing practices are urgently needed, Krever affirmed. And doctors, who should inform patients of the risks, benefits, and alternatives to transfusions, must exercise greater caution when using blood products, he said.

Krever addressed one of the biggest lapses in the blood system by calling upon the Red Cross and hospitals to do a better job of tracking down and notifying patients at risk from HIV and hepatitis C. Doctors should routinely ask both new and old patients about their past history with blood and blood products. He also called for expansion of the autologous blood program so patients facing elective surgery can store their own blood. And he recommended that some thought be given to "appropriate relief" for those infected in the future by contaminated blood. But these are just first steps to reform.

What happened to the hundreds of Canadians infected by HIV reflects the least redeeming features of human beings caught in a web of power struggles and secretive bureaucracy: arrogance on the part of the Red Cross national officers, sluggishness at a time of peril on the part of the Bureau of Biologics, ignorance on the part of some doctors, lack of leadership by government, the chase for dollars by manufacturers, and apathy and fear on the part of consumers. All played a role in the nightmare. Those who were entrusted with the obligation to protect blood and its users failed to respond in a timely way. They neglected to undertake tough measures required to ensure safety. They proved resistant to emerging new ideas and ignored advice that countered their narrow vision of the blood system. And they failed the test of leadership, only grudgingly agreeing to an investigation into how the system had failed.

If a thousand Canadians died after poisonous gas escaped from an aging chemical plant, or were killed when four fully loaded airliners collided at Pearson airport, there would be a hue and cry for an immediate and full inquiry. And so there should be. But when more than a thousand people faced death from contaminated blood, it took eight years to start an investigation. Even then, it did not happen until some courageous individuals spoke out, captured the public's attention, and won the ear of sympathetic politicians.

The tragic aftermath of tainted blood is reflected today in the faces of the recipients who are still living and the survivors of those who have died—Bill and Rita Marche, James Kreppner, Gloria Smith, Denise Orieux, Marlene and Jerry Freise, and all the others.

These people, and the families and friends whose lives have been damaged by the tragedy of bad blood, want the assurance that their agonizing experience will never be repeated. From their pain, we must hope that lessons have been learned and Canada's blood system in particular, and its health system in general, will be more responsive to the needs of those who depend on it. Future threats must be taken seriously and not brushed off by technocrats. Hemophiliacs infected with HIV and hepatitis C and other transfused victims make up a small percentage of Canadians, but they have been a red warning flag, showing us that the system was failing. And they remain a disconcerting reminder of shortcomings yet to be addressed.

We try to rationalize the fate of so many people by saying the guardians of the blood system and of the health system were only doing their best. We watch the haunting parade of survivors testify at the Krever inquiry, and know there are scores more who never had the chance to speak their piece. We know there are many deaths to come—some will be people we love. We witness power games and denial and finger-pointing every step of the way. There's a refusal to acknowledge that mistakes were made; a refusal to accept that consumers of health services have a right—indeed, a responsibility—to participate fully in the system, a refusal by the decision-makers to say they are genuinely sorry. When you talk with those who have been victimized, so many say the healing could begin if they received an official apology.

The minority of severe hemophiliacs who mistrusted the health system largely escaped the most dire consequences, while those who believed that the system would look after their needs were the ones who suffered most. "I don't feel anger now, or at any time, really," remarked John Wilson in the fall of 1993. "I feel a sense of betrayal. We have been betrayed by the system." For many others the trust that once existed has been replaced by unquenchable anger.

This erosion of trust may be the key to what we as a nation must learn from the tainted blood scandal. Medicine needs to be de-mystified so that citizens can become more active in how the medical system operates. Health consumers must always be on guard against complacency, convenience, financial short-cuts, and errors of judg-ment. And institutions that determine the quality and safety of our health care must be made accountable. Clearly, we have a long way to go.

KEY DATES

July 1982	Bruce Evatt of the Atlanta Centers for Disease Control warns that hemophiliacs would be prime candidates to develop the new syndrome.
August 1982	The Canadian Bureau of Biologics asks doctors and clinics to watch for AIDS cases among hemophiliacs.
October 1982	Drs. Hanna Strawczynski and Chris Tsoukas begin studies of the immune systems of Montreal hemophiliacs.
January 1983	Celebrated outburst by Don Francis of Atlanta Centers for Disease Control about how many hemophiliacs have to die before something is done.
	National Hemophilia Foundation in United States holds meeting on treatment procedures in light of AIDS. Attended by John Derrick of the Canadian Red Cross; Dr. Strawczynski, medical advisor to Canadian Hemophilia Society; and Dr. Tsoukas.
March 1983	The first Canadian hemophiliac dies of AIDS. Proof emerges that AIDS is caused by a virus. Medical advisors to the Canadian Hemophilia Society urge caution in use of concentrates.
May 1983	Dr. Roslyn Herst of Red Cross, also chair of the Ontario medical advisors, calls for treatment as usual.
November 1983	Heat-treated concentrates produced by the U.S. firm Baxter-Hyland are licensed for Canadian use.

January 1984	Report in the *Annals of Internal Medicine* says there is "substantial evidence that transfusion-related AIDS does occur."
July 1984	John Derrick's article in the *Canadian Medical Association Journal* downplays infection through blood.
Summer 1984	Michael O'Shaughnessy, training in the United States, finds that the majority of blood samples from Canadian hemophiliacs are HIV-infected.
September 1984	The medical journal *Lancet* publishes article stating that heat treating kills the HIV virus in concentrates.
Fall 1984	Pressure rises in Canada from several sources for use of heat-treated products. Both the federal Bureau of Biologics and the Red Cross doubt heat treatment is effective.
November 13, 1984	Cutter Laboratories heat-treated product is licensed for Canadian use.
November 16, 1984	The Bureau of Biologics calls for use of heat-treated products only.
December 6, 1984	A letter in the *New England Journal of Medicine* by Dr. Tsoukas suggests the majority of Canadian hemophiliacs are infected.
December 10, 1984	A consensus meeting is held under the direction of the Canadian Blood Committee, which gives medical advisors of Hemophilia Society the responsibility of determining which hemophiliacs get priority for heat-treated products.
January 1985	The Canadian Red Cross orders heat-treated products, a month and a half after federal regulator calls for its use exclusively.
April 25, 1985	First heat-treated products arrive at Red Cross.
May 1, 1985	First heat-treated products distributed.

July 1, 1985	Heat-treated products only are now to be distributed. Non-heated are to be recalled.
August 1, 1985	ELISA testing of blood donations approved by provinces.
September 1985	Some provinces start ELISA testing.
November 1, 1985	ELISA testing started in all provinces.
Fall 1987	Late HIV infections reported in Western Canada. Armour dry-heated products implicated.
August 1988	Canadian Hemophilia Society appeals for federal compensation.
December 14, 1989	Health Minister Perrin Beatty announces federal compensation of $30,000 a year for a maximum of four years for hemophiliacs and blood-transfused.
April 1, 1993	Final payment from federal compensation.
April 14, 1993	Nova Scotia health minister George Moody announces talks on provincial assistance.
May 1993	Commons sub-committee on health issues releases report.
September 15, 1993	Provincial assistance and inquiry announced.
February 14, 1994	Krever inquiry starts hearings.
March 15, 1994	Final date to sign waiver for provincial assistance.
June 1994	Canadian Hospital Association announces campaign to urge anyone who received a blood transfusion between 1978 and 1985 to be tested for HIV.
Summer 1994	Red Cross regional centres fail U.S. Food and Drug Administration inspections. Shipments of Canadian-source plasma to the United States halted.
February 24, 1995	Krever inquiry interim report.
December 1995	Deadline for Krever inquiry.

INDEX

104055